GUNGI BLUES

By Sanchita Islam

'One million people commit suicide every year'
The World Health Organization

Sanchita Islam

Published by
Chipmunkapublishing
PO Box 6872
Brentwood
Essex CM13 1ZT
United Kingdom

http://www.chipmunkapublishing.com

Edited by Sarah Broughton

GUNGI BLUES

Dedication

I wrote this book for my mother and late father in an attempt to try and visualise and recreate a world that existed before I was born.

GUNGI BLUES

Foreword

The idea to write Gungi Blues landed in my head when I was 21. I started to sketch out a few ideas and began in earnest at 23 to pen my first novel knowing all too well that I wasn't really the writer in the family. In fact I only started writing when my middle sister refused to realise her talent. I then abandoned the book and wrote another entitled 'Beautiful Boy,' at 24, only to return to Gungi Blues the following year. An editor Leo Hollis, who was working for Fourth Estate at the time, picked up the raw manuscript and wanted to take it on. Lacking in confidence I followed his every word amending the book and fashioning it to his tastes only for the book to be dropped a year later. At 27 I shelved the project and published a series of five books in the interim only to return to it many years later in 2005 when I was the grand old age of 32. I began to fiddle with the manuscript and at 33 I bumped into a publisher, Simon Prosser at Hamish Hamilton Penguin and a literary agent Sugra Zaman from Watson Little. They both liked the book and my confidence was restored but they said it needed some tweaking. So I began the torturous process of tearing the book apart only for Simon to say he wasn't interested after all and for Sugra to say she was going to have a baby and that unfortunately since she was leaving I would be dropped from Watson Little.

After this I simply wanted to incinerate both versions since neither really came close to what I originally planned to write in fact the very first manuscript that I showed to Leo has vanished, well I probably misplaced or chucked it.

Now I am in the lucky position to be signed with a publisher that doesn’t give a toss what the establishment thinks but after everything I have been through I am ambivalent about this book and still think it is ‘rubbish.’ However, Rachel Lichtenstein, author of ‘On Brick Lane’ and the scholar Elisabetta Marino, lecturer in English at Rome Tor Vergata University, are both fans of the book. This is what they said:

‘A compelling, beautifully written novel, which has the power to unsettle every stereotypical perception and totally involve the reader.’ (Elisabetta Marino, Rome Tor Vergata University)

‘Sanchita Islam is a highly talented artist, writer and film maker whose creative output knows no end. Having been a fan of her artwork for many years I was delighted to read her first major novel, 'Gungi Blues', which in my opinion represents the authentic voice of the Bangladeshi Diaspora in Britain today. I think it's a very powerful story with an authentic feel about it and a fresh voice … I have no doubt it will be a great success.’ (Rachel Lichtenstein, author On Brick Lane and Rodinski’s Room)

So, if two of my respected and dear colleagues enjoyed the book I hope you do to. The version that I have decided to publish is not the mashed up ‘Penguin’ pleasing version but the mashed up ‘Fourth Estate’ pleasing version. I just wish I could find the original manuscript!

GUNGI BLUES

Gungi –A gungi is a word that my mother used when I was small. She never told me what it meant. It is pronounced 'Gung – ee.' If you were to call someone a gungi it would imply that the person is a mad, unconventional person, with a unique view on life. This story is a tale of one family's gungi blues.

Sanchita Islam

GUNGI BLUES

1979 Manchester

'Bastard child, I wish you were never born' screamed Mina, her eyes bulging, her hair in splinters, her face screwed up in wrinkles.

Ana remembered accidentally kicking her sister up the putki; they were just playing and her knee sort of slipped. Rimi bent over double wincing in pain. She was incredibly apologetic although Ana couldn't quite contain her giggles. Mina walked in and demanded to know what had happened. When Rimi whimpered the story and Mina saw the smirk that stained Ana's face she seized her pink feather duster and started whacking her daughter across her bare thigh. Ana tried to run away from her but tripped and landed in a heap at the bottom of the stairs. Mina stood over Ana, flaring her nostrils. She looked like a terrifying tough super human baddie. Bracing herself, Ana covered her head and prepared for another serious dosage of whacking. She saw Mina's hand pluck a long thin plastic thing that lay dormant by the radiator and heard the rustle of her silk sari as she held her hand high before attacking the same spot of leg with the force of a warrior. She stopped hitting Ana after a while but she could still hear her heavy breathing. Ana didn't move and her arms remained firmly wrapped around her head until the sound of Mina's shrill voice made Ana jump. Nervously Ana wiped away the dribble that laced her chin with a shirt sleeve. Mina told Ana to get up, called her a 'haramsada', which means bastard in Bangla, and to stop crying because she hadn't hit her that hard. Numb from pain, Ana sat up slowly and peered down at her leg. The skin was swelling a candyfloss pink in a nice stripy pattern across Ana's outer thigh. Ana watched, with a perverse fascination, as the stripes began to bulge with a soft soreness and she paused before slowly limping upstairs to her room to sob discreetly in a pillow.

Ana lived in a cramped semi-detached house on 6 Whitebrook Road in Fallowfield, Manchester. The house stood on a long row of houses with neat front gardens lined with pretty flowers that matched the curtains. That is apart from Ana's. Their garden was usually unkempt, dotted with dandelions, the hedge-row wonky, the gate covered in an abstract pattern of yellowed, hardened bird shit, the windows streaky from black paint that flaked messily onto the concrete paving and the rose bushes were wild sprawling things that gave birth to pink, white and yellow blooms. Ana always wondered why Miss Redfern, their nice grey haired neighbour, had grass that looked like lush green velvet and poppies, a deeper shade of blood.

Miss Redfern perennially re-painted her house the same shade of olive. The colour of the house was the only way to distinguish one from the next. Mrs Harrison, who lived opposite, painted her house in cool emeralds that blended with her potted ferns. Every Friday she played Black Jack with old Jim and in her green house she grew tomatoes, which she gave as gifts to the neighbours. They were the colour of peas and hard but with some salt and lemon juice they tasted all right. Miss Redfern and Mrs Harrison were two of the ubiquitous old ladies that lived on Whitebrook Road.

Mrs Ballwinkle at number nine was seventy-two. She seldom left her house and kept her curtains drawn. Occasionally, Ana glimpsed the old lumpy figure through her bedroom window creaking down in her lilac dressing gown for her one-pint of milk before slipping back inside for hibernation.

Mr and Mrs Walsh were an Irish couple that lived in the next semi down the road. Mrs Walsh had white fluffy hair and always wore navy linen dresses. In their front room the only thing hanging on the wall was an elaborate family tree spanning six generations of Walsh's. Their house wasn't particularly tidy. They allowed the grass to grow just beyond its borders before dragging out the lawn mower. In the summer Mr Walsh mowed the lawn in a greyish string vest and his pale shoulders would turn a shiny pink with sweat and sunburn.

Auntie Pat lived in the only detached house on Whitebrook Road. She possessed a soft reclining chair in her back garden and a sun bed in the spare room. Auntie Pat was the youngest of the neighbours at fifty-nine, but looked older than her years with skin prematurely wrinkled from years of sun worship and too many fags. There were scores of other people who lived on Whitebrook road but Ana only recognised their rockeries, the type of car in the driveway, or the colour of their door. It was a street full of people walking their dogs, trimming their hedge-ways or sitting by their windows.

Once Ana saw a young couple rendez-vous outside Mrs Harrison's house. They had a secret snog and then disappeared down the street. She rarely saw any other kids apart from a pair of Asian families that lived in the row of houses facing the back garden. Both families lived in two houses but treated them as one. Between them they had four kids who resembled one another and played together in their joined up back garden. Ana remembered watching them tie their pet Alsation to a tree and then take turns kicking its head in.

Beyond Whitebrook Road was the main road, the road that stemmed into Wilmslow Road, the road that led to Oxford Road and Manchester town centre. On Wilmslow Road was the Swiss bakery that sold chocolate éclairs and cinnamon buns; the Jabberwocky, a former church renovated into a bar to cater for the students that lived in the beige blocks of Owens Park; Malcolm Bishop, filled with elephant mobiles, fancy pens, Birthday cards and pretty hand painted useless things; and the Canadian Charcoal Pit that made burgers with whole chunks of gherkin and piles of fried onion rings. On a side street behind the Jabberwocky was a butcher's store run by a Bangladeshi man called Tariq. He was a small, skinny man with a thick moustache that filled half his face. His girlfriend was blond and taller than him. She would often be left waiting in his battered white van listening to Timmy Malik on the radio. Lining his shelves were dusty packets of Rice Krispies, jars of Coleman's mustard, toilet roll and an array of other goods that became permanent features of decoration. The shop smelt of sour meat and the floor was covered in soiled bits of animal. Tariq minced beef on the spot and gave away free chicken legs to regular customers; that's why there was always a queue. Then there was the Newsagents at the top of the road. An old couple that never had kids ran it; they had a Chihauhau instead. They dressed him in a tartan jacket and tied his silky hair in ribbons. He barked like mad and scared Ana but he always kept his place under the counter in the shop. The couple boasted an impressive sweetie counter; Half penny Cola Fizzes, Flying Saucers, Black Jacks, Banana Chews and Bon Bons. And, if Ana was skint and fancied something substantial there were home made Vimto lollies at tuppence each.

Fallowfield was Ana's neighbourhood and 6 Whitebrook Road was her first home. Ana's house was a tiny miny house. Downstairs, was a yellow kitchen with marble patterned work-tops covered in clutter, a living room with stained sofas concealed under cheap material, a front room with nice clean sofas and a fake Rodin. Upstairs, there was a tiny blue toilet, a bathroom with chipped tiles, Ana's parents' room was crammed with a dressing table inhabited with Estee Lauder lotions and used tissue clumps, another bedroom with a nasty brown patterned linoleum floor and a brown carpeted room they called the ‘small room’. The house was bursting with plants, an Ivy in the hall, a Money plant hanging on the wall, a Cheese plant in the living room, potted Begonias and Fuchsias at every turn. With plants in each room, even the tiny loo, their house became a living organism crawling with leaves that sucked up the light, stretching stems that inhabited the walls and dead bits that eventually congealed into the flower patterned carpet. Then there was the back garden, overgrown with giant weeds and a bent swing. Beside it was a garage stuffed with boxes of rubbish and in a bag, under a broken chair, were old porno mags left by the previous occupant.

This was Ana’s house where she lived with her two sisters Rimi and Bela, her father Amit Bai and mother Mina.

GUNGI BLUES

The Other World

Mina came to Manchester from another world.

A green, moist, dry, dusty world with cracked concrete roads, half-naked kids, spitting old women and men pissing in ponds covered in leafy duvets.

Pathuakali was Mina's district, a small district in Bangladesh.

Manchester 1999

In 1984 Mina and Amit Bai moved from Fallowfield to Didsbury, the posh bit of Manchester. They never visited Whitebrook Road again.

Mr Walsh: dead
Cause of death: He was mowing the lawn one sunny afternoon and had a stroke. Amit Bai found him lying face down in the garden. An ambulance came and took him away. After that Mrs Walsh let the grass grow and grow. She died a few years later.

Mrs Harrison: dead
Cause of death: She stopped going out in the garden as the Alzheimer's robbed her, very slowly first, of the need; the need to check her green tomatoes, the need to play black jack, the need to say hello, to breathe, to live.

Auntie Pat: dead
Cause of death: lung cancer from too many fags that she refused to ever give up.

Mrs Ballwinkle: dead
Cause of death: stroke. This little old lady was the first to die on the street but she was waiting for her time to leave many years before.

Miss Redfern: dead
Cause of death: It was a slow burn for Miss Redfern; she was the last to die. She lived as a

spinster all her life, she didn't change the way she dressed, she didn't change the colour of her door and she never missed Wimbledon until she started to wet herself. At first she cleaned up the mess but then it became uncontrollable. Her house began to reek and she began to forget and as the decay set in the house started to rot. Mina heard about the incontinence and decided to visit Miss Redfern. No one ever imagined that Miss Redfern would grow old and frail. She was the horse who carried three Asda shopping bags in one fist. When Miss Redfern opened the door, her face was gaunt and saggy with wrinkles. She barely recognised Mina until she mentioned the children's names. Miss Redfern ushered Mina into her house. It was dirty and smelt of old people's urine. The frail thin thing hobbled with a walking stick. She had fallen on the hard pavement and broken her leg some months ago. Her health had never been the same since. As Mina reminisced about the good times Miss Redfern looked lost like a child. The old memories were fading and Miss Redfern was rotting in a pit of loneliness. The sickness and stink was too much to swallow. Miss Redfern hobbled to the door and they stood on the doorstep for a little while. Mina noticed the front garden. It was overgrown now. The rose bushes strangled with weeds. The shrubs withered. The flowerbeds dry. When Miss Redfern was finally admitted to hospital Mina never visited. She died a few months later, alone.

Sanchita Islam

Drawing Mina 1999

There was a heap of newspapers on the dirty cream carpet. Old Manchester Evening News and stray Sunday Times supplements. A cotton bud, yellow at either end, a book left open spilling Bangla text and a lady snoring in bed. Must have been four, maybe five o'clock in the afternoon? Curtains drawn, lamp on. Chapped lips slightly open. Freckles hiding in the folds of her neck. Egg whites peeping through the slits of her lids. Spider's nest of black hair. Tufts trapped in a sandwich of skin. A twitch of an over plucked brow. And fifty odd years of angst stuck in a frown.

With her pinpoint pencil Ana wanted to continue the ritual of drawing her mother that began years ago when she was eleven. Felt tip red lips, silver blotches for pearls, blue pencil eye shadow and HB grey curly hair. Eight and a half out of ten, that's what Mrs Allen, the art teacher, gave Ana. Looking back the drawing was far too small, her mother's neck too short, eyes too big, lips too pouty, hair too curly and pearls too silver, but it wasn't bad for an eleven year old. Now, fifteen years later, she sat armed with HBs, 8Bs, 2Bs and sharpened lumps of graphite. Poised to etch out her mother's face from nothing, Ana smoothed out the white of the paper. Was there anything more perfect than a white piece of paper? The paper was whiter than white. Even smelt white if white possessed a smell. The white calmed her in a world where there was nothing but mess. Postcards of men in boats sailing the rivers of Bangladesh stuck to the door. Empty Estee

GUNGI BLUES

Lauder bottles stacked up on the dressing table. Cracks in the walls, mould on the ledge, condensation on the windows, a pink elephant with only one ear by the bed. Any space was crammed with something apart from that piece of paper.

It was always the same. Ana had to beg Mina to draw her. She would lie there and grumble under the covers sliding between the now and the memories locked in her head.

'No,' she'd say angrily.

'Don't poke me, you are always poking me.'

'I'm not poking you; I just want to draw you.'

'Leave me alone,' Ana looked up at Amit Bai. He was lying in bed. His glasses were propped on the tip of his Roman nose. His teeth lay in a white plastic box on the bedside table and he was scratching his head as he read the paper.

'Stop it, you'll go bald,' Mina snapped. Amit Bai carried on itching.

'Why won't she let me draw her?'

Amit Bai gave Mina one of his hard looks 'Don't be mean, sit for her.'

Mina was lying on her back. The hairs from her plait escaped into a wild orgy on her head. She was wearing her old pink night dress. Ana could make out her left breast. She worked out the size of her brown nipple through the faded pink. Tufts of black arm-pit hair jutted out, from under soft skin. Her shoulders were slightly dimpled; arms still smooth and hair free, hands a little worn from too much washing up without gloves. Mina didn't have any hard skin on the soles of her feet and hardly any hair on her legs apart from a few spidery strays on her ankle. Ana watched Mina's toes wiggle themselves into a frenzy. Mina peered out from under the duvet, like a child, and seeing Ana sitting, waiting, hoping she shouted 'get lost' and reassembled herself in her warm cave.

Amit Bai continued to scratch his head. Mina retreated further and her body became one big mole hill. She heard Ana pack up her pencils and get up to go. Ana was almost through the door when Mina pushed back the covers and looked up shyly.

'OK then you can draw me,' she said in a baby voice. Almost instantly she was grumpy again.

'Why do you always draw me? Why don't you draw him?'

'He's not as interesting as you.'

'Don't try and flatter me you cheeky.'

GUNGI BLUES

'You should draw her fat arse.' Amit Bai cackled, Mina pinched his cheek and he let out a fake yelp that made her giggle. Ana was laughing hard. A special laughter that came from the gut, a laughter that was real and made Ana's belly ache.

A spot light lit up Mina's face. She was frowning. It wasn't an ordinary frown. It was like a deep dark cut that split her forehead into two halves. Her eyes creased up into little quivering lines. Freckles too many to count. Nose slightly dry on the tip. Lips leaking out like the bulge of a belly. Ana observed every nuance in her mother's face and tried to capture the strange unfathomable creature that lay before her. A gentle snore kept Ana company until Mina winced.

'Have you finished? I'm in so much pain.'

'Just a little longer,' Ana lied,

'Why do you torture me? I'm not your specimen,' she said.

Ana was too busy hacking to care about her pain. She started with the heavy lids first, then a thick line of lashes that guided Ana to the dark circles, creased and black, to the complex furrows of a brow that constantly moved as Mina tried to settle into a reluctant sleep. Ana knew she was still awake because her eyes were twitching with the weight of a dead past. Mina started to murmur. Started to tell Ana stories. Stories that she repeated over the years. Ana had heard them all before and sometimes she would groan 'change the tape.' It was if that old tape was stuck in her head. Mina never changed it. She just rewound it and played it over and over. And Ana listened as Mina would talk about that 'other world' where she was born and twitch her feet as she travelled back.

GUNGI BLUES

The Pink House

Mina's house was painted pastel pink and modest in structure. Mud kitchen at the back, gas burner for a stove and a small pond full of snakes that slithered up legs, this was the house in Bangladesh where Mina lived. With her seven siblings and parents Nana and Nanu, they shared three rooms with a pet chicken that roamed under the bed.

Tall with wispy white beard and thick-rimmed glasses that slipped down his nose when he read the paper, Nana woke up at 5 a.m. each morning to the cawing of crows. Waiting for him on his side table was a glass of lemon juice. Every day he drank the juice of several lemons believing that his skin would remain fair and soft like mashed potato. And every day Nana fiddled with his mat before muttering, kneeling and raising his hands with rhythmic precision while Nanu performed her ritual of standing in the kitchen prodding Nana's egg with a spoon. Diminutive with black wavy hair, button nose, Thai almond eyes, Slovenian cheekbones, Jamaican juicy lips and English schoolgirl freckles, she looked something of a hybrid; the product of a sexual liaison between a Burmese maid and her Arab master.

Heating sand until it hissed, Nanu tossed rice onto the smoking golden bed, watching the grains pop and jump, expanding into fat white maggots of Khoy, before scattering them in pretty patterns on a dollop of home made yoghurt.

Squatting in his corner, Dolu, their old manservant, slowly sliced mango, banana and papaya onto a plate, sneaking stray slithers into his mouth while licking the sweet syrup from his bony fingers.

Nana was sitting at his desk surrounded by mounds of papers, old receipts and stray taka. Dolu emerged with an overladen tray and Nana happily distracted himself with food. The mango, a brilliant orange, tasted slightly over ripe. The banana, brown around the edges, too sweet. The papaya, anaemic and hard like boiled potato. Disappointed he tried the cereal. Nicely crisp and still warm, he forgave the lack lustre selection of fruit and wolfed down the rest in a few spoonfuls. Unaware that his whiskers were painted in yoghurt, he gathered his papers and set off for work with his brow furrowed deep, wondering what Nanu would make him for lunch.

Nana sat in his spacious civil servants office furnished with three desks and a cabinet that he shared with his two elderly colleagues. He could have moved to the city with his qualifications but in Dhaka he would have been like a mosquito among millions all sucking from the same corpse. His crinkly white bearded colleagues wrote furiously with heads' bent low over dusty desks. Nana wrote a few letters in English, filed several papers, sharpened his pencil, tidied his desk and then watched the minutes tick by on the clock above the filing cabinet.

GUNGI BLUES

Ana tried to picture Nana's world as Mina described it; she'd met him twice in Bangladesh. She remembered his wispy elegant beard and his gentle voice. His skin was smooth and youthful. Mina would talk of his temper and Ana found it hard to believe. How could this dignified old man be such a monster? Ana wanted to preserve her own image of Nana, still clear in her mind: tall, fair, kind and beautiful.

They ate dinner by eight o'clock; Nana always expected his food to be ready on time. Nanu and Dolu assembled the final dishes. Fish glistening in sauces made with a secret blend of spices. Chicken nestling with potatoes so soft they fell apart with a nudge. Pulses and beans fried and boiled. Dhal dressed in coriander. Rice that was fluffy and light as a cloud. And salad that sat like an intricate mosaic in a glass bowl.

Seated crossed legged on the floor everyone watched Nanu fill Nana's plate before he raised a hand to stop the onslaught of fish gravy. Moulding salad, dhal, rice and fish into a perfect ball Nana took his first chew. His face screwed up like a prune and the mood changed from serenity to madness in half a second. Nana threw his plate across the room. It flew long and high, rather elegantly, in the air, before landing in a shattered mess of China fragments and flecks of golden fish. Flinching with the crash Mina didn't know where to look.

Backing into a corner Nana walked up to his wife and slapped her across the cheek. Hard. Hard enough for her lip to burst. A blob of blood trickled down her chin. With shaking beard and closed eyes, Nana ranted incoherently about food, salt and money. Taking a chance, Nanu slipped away to lock herself in the hut she called her kitchen. Following her outside, Nana banged on the door until his fists blushed pink. Still and quiet Nanu listened to his threats. Growing hysterical in the silence Nana kicked the door. Each kick shook Nanu's body to the core. The cold misery of fear crept through Nanu's body like bare feet running on ice but she didn't budge. Nana gave up after three minutes. With limp foot and a belly too empty to beat his wife he returned to his food, where Mina and her siblings sat like stone staring into shiny plates. Sinking to the floor Nana ordered everyone to 'eat'.

Two hours later Nanu re-emerged to collect dirty dishes and caught the low murmur of Nana's drifting prayer.

'Please forgive me Allah for my temper...' he muttered over and over in feeble whispers.

Hearing these words. The shame. The guilt. Nanu pulled a face. A sour crinkled face. A face that had heard it all before.

Mina prayed that night too. She prayed for good food everyday. Food that melted in Nana's mouth and caressed his stomach. Food that left Nana content enough to retire to his room to read the paper. And in her dreams Mina saw Nanu trembling in the corner with blood on her face. Nana was screaming at her to get out before grabbing Nanu by the arm and pushing her out the house. Mina waited in her dream. Waited for Nanu to come back. She never did.

'Are you sure Nana did these things?' Ana asked quietly. Mina was locked in that 'other world' she didn't want to come back. She didn't answer, just mumbled on about being the 'middle' child. Ana delicately drew a thick line of lashes and listened.

Mina was the middle child, number four. Not too short and not too tall with a heart shaped face, big eyes like a cow, fat lips, Nanu's Burmese nose, two ice cream balls of flesh that sat on her cheekbones and skin the colour of varnished pine. She was born after a pair of twins.

'They were two beautiful boys. Bright eyed and button nosed. So beautiful they were. I still see their faces and hear their cries in my dreams.' Nanu pined.

Mina saw them too and most nights, particularly those sleepless, sore eyed nights when the mind refuses to stop, Mina whispered to herself: 'I wish I was a boy.'

'To be a boy was to be free' Mina believed. Her three brothers Omar, Babu and Moyd ran around the house in their underwear and climbed coconut trees in search of juice and white coconut flesh. But Nana openly preferred girls, Mina never new why. Nana sent all his children to school including his daughters. Mina and her sisters, Conna, Papri and Boo Boo studied up to secondary level. Nana employed personal tutors for them all.

Encouraging Mina to 'read, read, read until your brain is 'heavy', Nanu sat on the edge of the bed talking in whispers about the barbarism of Ghengis Khan and recited the poetry of Tagore. Letting the minutes slip by, Mina latched onto every word, like a kid sucking on sweets, as the others slept on.

Mina read under the bed, beneath the shade of a tree or at her tiny desk. When she showed her school reports to Nana he responded with a nod of approval while Nanu, although she gave Mina a rigorous pat on the head, always had a look in her eye; a look which said 'you can do even better.'

Nana never had any money. He was 'useless' financially Mina said. To pay her school fees Mina was forced to ask a distant acquaintance. He was actually more like a stranger. The one with tufts of hair that clung to the tips of his ear lobes like spiders. The one who lived in that big white house, decorated with lush plants and red flowers. The one that Nana said had 'money hidden in plant pots'. On her way home she often saw the tubby man sitting on his veranda, ready with a smile for her. To avoid those lips she developed a trick of breaking into a sprint just before reaching his house. That afternoon Mina didn't run. She looked around, there was a man crossing the other side of the street wearing a Hawaiian patterned shirt, a girl sitting on the ground playing in the dirt and a scrawny man carrying a pole lined with hanging, squawking chickens. The tubby man was standing in his doorway, and seeing her hovering, scuttled out to catch her. Mina asked hesitantly if she could borrow some money; he agreed without much need for persuasion and went off to get it. Mina waited in the hall way. It was cluttered with landscapes painted in lurid colours and gold pots that lined his tiled floor. Sliding into the bedroom he pulled out notes tucked away in secret corners and returned with a few torn taka. Mina stretched out her hand as the tubby man counted the money. He stood expectantly and, reluctantly, Ana edged towards the man's dome of a tummy avoiding the wet patches of his armpits. Wrapping her up in his arms and rubbing his hands over her cotton back his fingers began to creep under her shirt. Hard skin against soft. Clammy palms pressing deep. Crawling fingers searching for breast. Squeezing flesh. Gripping tight. Wriggling free Mina broke away. The tubby man laughed as if he'd heard a funny joke and said 'you are like a little fish.' Mina stared into his round face and open mouth. He stooped down and kissed her long and hard on the head. She was glad she hadn't washed her hair for three days. The tubby man escorted her to the door and as she walked down the mud path he waved and smiled that smile. The tears were already welling up. She had no control. Fat, hot, stinging tears rolled down her cheeks entertaining passing strangers. When she reached home Dolu didn't notice her puffy red eyes. Nanu didn't notice her lack of appetite at dinner. And when she lay in bed her body twitched with the pinch of fat creeping fingers in the dark.

Mina paid her school fees the next morning, just like all the other kids. She should have been happy but she wasn't smiling. During class she tried to concentrate but the words just drifted over images of the tubby man.

Ana wondered if the man had raped Mina and this was just a muted down version of the real story. She didn't say anything and scratched out black wisps of hair with a stick of graphite. Something inside Ana made her feel sick, that Mina had to ask that man for money, that Nana didn't take responsibility. There was something strangely familiar about the story, the innate feeling of insecurity, of feeling alone in the world.

Mina took the long route home through the forest. She observed the sprouting lotus that spread across the patches of green pond, the light that filtered through the leaves and paused to watch a toddler hack a coconut open with a machete. A low cacophony of birds, insects, wind and footsteps kept her company before a sharp sound from behind a bush startled her. A short skinny man wearing a checked lungi and Hawaiian patterned shirt appeared. The top buttons were left open, exposing a burst of thick black hair like the bristles of a hairbrush. His cheeks were pitted with holes gouged from picked mosquito bites and his forehead shimmered with a thin sheet of sweat. Flashing a cigarette stained grin, he walked cockily towards Mina until they were face to face and breathing heavily said

'I saw you go with that fat old man last night.'

She stared blankly into his face, thin and angular with a pointy nose and crusty lips.

'What do you want?' Mina asked unable to hide the little tremors of fear in her voice.

'Give me your hand?' He said calmly. Gripping it tight he began to rub her skinny wrist with his hard thumbs.

Mina felt nothing apart from a sweaty stickiness.

Her hand tensed up and as she tried to pull away he pushed her stiff fingers straight down on his bulge. Hard and lumpy through the thin cotton. Her fingers protested but he coerced them up and down. Pressing down. Panting like a dog. Fumbling with his lungi. Exposing his cock. Dark brown sticking out of a black bush. Mina jolted at the sight of it. The man grinned, getting off on the fear in her eyes, getting harder and harder.

Mina screamed. A scream that came from another place, deep within.

He let go for barely a second but it was enough. Mina started to run. She didn't look back she just ran. Standing half naked, with his lungi sitting at his ankles, the man didn't chase her, he just watched her stick legs shrink in the distance and shouted after her

'I know where you live.'

Sharp things buried themselves deep into her feet but still she ran. Running until her legs grew heavy and the pain of a stitch pricked her side like needles, she squatted by the stump of a tree, rocking back and forth with nothing but the sound of crickets to smudge out her fear and the shade of the spindly trees to keep her hidden. Legs covered in cuts and scratches. Feet dirty. School uniform torn. Walking in pin steps, finding any excuse to pause, she stumbled past familiar trees until her little pink house, the colour of sweet strawberry mousse, loomed in the distance. Dolu was dishing out cow shit in the yard, smoothing it out with his hands, too busy caressing the brown goo to notice her.

GUNGI BLUES

Mina traipsed off to the bedroom with head hung low. The gentle hum of breathing and Boo Boo's snoring made Ana felt safe in that tiny room. Her three sisters all lay snug under their covers, eyes slightly open, mouths dribbling. Mina sat on the edge of the bed and watched them. Minutes ticked by. Still she sat. A spider crawled into the low light of the candle and Ana watched the animal panic in the light. Ana edged closer and killed it with the edge of her palm, squashing it flat; she peeled off her clothes with stiff hands and climbed into bed, toe nails black with dirt, limbs creaking with ache. Deep in images, she saw the man in the Hawaiian shirt. His bad skin. Yellow teeth. Limp cock. Sweaty fingers. Over and over she saw him until the crows started to caw and light twinkled through the window.

A month passed during which Mina took funny routes home constantly looking over her shoulder, anticipating a chance encounter. She saw a short bald man in the street buying Chana Chor from a vendor but it wasn't the tubby man. She saw a man wearing a blue and pink shirt squatting by the side of the road rolling up a leaf of Paan but it wasn't the man in the Hawaiian shirt. She saw her assaulters in the faces of strangers. They sat there consuming her thoughts, invading those quiet seldom moments, hijacking her dreams and there was nothing she could do.

It was afternoon. The sun was on its way down casting a blanket of light that made everything look brand new and made Mina squint and sweat. She walked with a stoop, her bag overloaded with too many books. Dolu saw her struggling in the distance and waved happily at her. The strap of her bag sank into her fleshy shoulder and the sight of pink made her quicken pace. Mina enjoyed the breeze when rickshaw drivers raced past. She headed for the house, brushing passed Papri in the dirt yard, before a familiar voice forced her to stop. That's when she saw him sitting with Nana, happily guzzling from a bowl swimming with three creamy balls of roshaguli.

It was the tubby man, eating with his mouth open, joking with Nana, slapping him on the back, calling him 'brother.'

"You know, Baiya, my wife's getting old and the children have all grown up now." said the tubby man changing tone slightly.

'Your wife's not old,' replied Nana.

"The thing is, Baiya, I really want to get married again."

'Do you?' said Nana curiously.

'You see the reason why I came round was because I'm interested in one of your daughters. The middle one, the one with the wavy hair and freckles. What's her name again?' he asked screwing up his face.

GUNGI BLUES

Nana shuffled in his chair and tried to hide his feelings behind a breaking voice.

'My daughter's not ready for marriage.'

'She's ripe for marriage.'

'I don't think so.'

"Why not?"

'You're over forty, she's only fifteen.

'Fifteen's not so young. You know my cousin, he's fifty and he's onto his third wife. The lucky bastard just bagged himself a fourteen-year-old beauty'

Nana's beard began to shake.

'I'd rather drown my daughter in the river than let you marry her.'

The tubby man's smile faded, and as he got up to leave he said with a sly grin

'Oh, Baiya, before I forget could you please remind that daughter of yours about the taka I lent her. Thank you for the tea and roshaguli' and then he left.

Mina wanted to melt into the shadows as she watched Nana's face turn a paler shade of white. She tried to slip away but Nana glimpsed her hovering in the corner.

'Did you ask for money from that fat man?' Erupted Nana.

Mina stayed quiet.

'Did you?'

She caved in to the tremors of his voice.

'I'm sorry Abu but I knew you didn't have the money and I had to pay my school fees.' She whispered. 'I was going to pay the money back...'

Nana walked up to Mina and shouted millimetres from her face, close enough for her to feel the splinters of spit attack her skin. She clutched her bag of books for comfort but Nana ripped the bag from her hands.

'All this education is a bloody waste of time and money. I should just marry you off to that fat man. That's all you're good for.' He shouted as he emptied the contents of her bag onto the floor and kicked books, pencil case and pens across the room. Mina watched as her things received a battering before Nana paused to pick up a notebook that lay safe under the table and began to tear it, page by page, under her nose.

GUNGI BLUES

'Please Abu, stop it,' protested Mina in a whimpering voice.

'Chuup.'

Nana cut her short with a clean slap across the cheek. A slap that made her head shake. Her skin began to sting like nettles. She didn't rub her cheek better, she didn't bawl her eyes out, she just stood with her eyes glued to the floor and tried to avoid the mess of broken pencils, tattered books and ripped up papers at her feet.

'Taking money from strangers, Have you no shame? You're no better than a common whore.'

With a face twisted in a mess of lines and wrinkles, nasty things continued to spew out Nana's mouth and each word pricked her like the sharp bite of a mosquito. Mina slowly retreated to the bedroom. The sound of deep snores and smacking lips of her siblings irritated her as she undressed. When her head hit the pillow silent tears fell from her twisted face and her body shook with violent sobs. She became numb and her numbness turned into a seething something. Not anger, something else - hot and violent.

'I shit on them. I shit on them all,' she whispered over and over as some form of comfort.

When she closed her eyes she entered a world where she was shouting back at Nana. , screaming at him until she saw fear in his eyes. She was jumping up and down on that tubby man's head, like a trampoline, until bits of his brain got stuck in between her toes. She was tying the man in the Hawaiian shirt to a coconut tree, cutting his penis off with a rusty old knife and planting it in the dirt to rot.

Mina woke up the next morning to hear Nana shouting for Dolu in the background. She got out of bed, eyes sore from animated sleep, and dragged her feet to the toilet with a stoop. Nana emerged from his room and when he saw Mina he glared at her. A glare that stung her deep, like a nasty burn and then he looked away. At breakfast Mina watched as he stroked Boo Boo's hair with tender fingers and invited her two younger brothers to accompany him to the market. His eyes glazed over her as if she didn't exist and for seven days Mina was like a stranger, a moving shadow, a thing in the corner until Nana broke the silence with a casual voice:

'Can you send this letter to the post office?'

Mina was stunned for a moment but she gladly took the letter from Nana and ran to the post office, arriving out of breath. On her way home people noticed her smile, her lively walk and bouncing black locks. And for half a second all the stuff in her head seemed like a silly blip, a speck of dust, a pin point dot because Nana was talking to her again.

Mina walked in to find Nana sitting in the main room reading the paper. Mina sat opposite him expecting something. But there was nothing. No explanation, no forgive and forget embrace, no glance, no nod, no grump, no sound. After five minutes of waiting Mina just left. She slumped on her bed and pulled out a book from a shelf lined with many. She turned the pages for the sake of turning. She was barely digesting; her mind was elsewhere wondering why Nana blanked her. Why he was up and down like a temperamental yo-yo. Why his smile mutated into a scowl and his laughter shifted smoothly into screams. To flush out thoughts trapped in a small hole in her head she surrendered to the words on the page, gorging on them until she felt sick.

Reading became her ritual.

The thing she did every day without fail. Sitting alone in the library while the other kids chatted and gossiped, she copied passages out of books in perfect joined up writing. Squatting in the bedroom corner, swaying on tiptoe, she memorised other people's words. Words rescued her from the tubby man's sugary smile. Words distracted her from imaginary fingers crawling up skirts. Words temporarily erased cocks, fingers and ranting fathers. Formulae sent her to sleep and she began to memorise futile facts such as the surface area of the inside of a lung is the size of a large pond.

Mina developed a predilection for juicy biological detail. A taste for dissecting locusts, disembodying delicate limbs and tearing up internal organs. It was during these heavy dissection sessions that she realised she wanted to be a doctor. When she tentatively broached the subject of studying medicine, one Sunday morning over chapattee and aloo, Nana replied 'you can't study at medical school?'

'Why not?'

'It's full of boys and you know what boys are like, they're always up to naughty giddy.'

Bemused, Mina asked 'So what should I study then?'

'Anything you like without boys.'

Eager to continue her education she ended up studying Chemistry exclusively with girls at Dhaka University and returned home during the holidays. After completing her degree Mina received a place to do her Msc in Bio Chemistry. Nana was relieved when she was awarded a scholarship. Papri, Conna and Boo Boo did not go onto university. They stayed at home. Papri helped Nanu with the chores, Conna chased boys and Boo Boo spent much of her time admiring her reflection in any shiny surface. The three sisters were waiting for marriage, their only escape route from home. Mina had other plans. She wanted to get a job, work and see the world beyond Bangladesh.

The drawing was complete and Mina was finally deep in sleep. Ana wondered what life would have been like if Mina had achieved her childhood dream and become a doctor. Ana couldn't picture her mother getting up early and tending to the sick and needy. Listening to the woes of patients, prescribing pills and checking blood pressure. Not Mina. Not this woman lying before her. She stared at her mother and wondered why she was this eccentric, plant loving, rabbit worshipping, scatty thing; why she was agnostic when her siblings never missed a prayer; why she was so messy and walked around in her night dress most days, not bothering to even brush her hair; why she was she so different; why she was this woman? Ana inspected the drawing, Mina looked at least twenty years older. Every line in her face was magnified, every blemish, every wrinkle. On that paper Ana saw a frightened old woman weighed down with apprehension and melancholy. Each drawing was the same, Mina sleeping, mouth slightly open, frowning, hair in a mess. And after executing one drawing Ana wanted to start another and another. It was her ritual; her way of trying to unravel Mina through shading and cross hatching, rather than words.

Mina was whispering a name in her sleep. Boo Boo. She was always talking about Boo Boo, her eldest sister. The last time Ana saw Boo Boo she was old and haggard with powdered white cheeks and a moustache like Salvador Dali. But Mina and Amit Bai still referred to Boo Boo as the great beauty of the family. She was the fairest of the four sisters with pearl skin, thick black hair wavy from plaiting, plump pink lips, arched cheekbones, and eyes the colour of burnt toast. Each night she spent at least one hour sitting before a cracked mirror widening her eyes with a thick line of black and whitening her cheeks with talcum powder. Mina compared the colour of her skin with her sister's, wondering why she was the colour of blemished wheat.

'I wish I was fair like you,' she whispered.

Bora Kala dusted Mina's cheeks with talc. Mina looked at the two white patches on her cheeks. She looked like a clown, a beggar with a pigmentation disorder, anything but beautiful.

Over the next few weeks Nana addressed the question of marrying off his eldest daughter. First there was the issue of suitability. Occupation, level of education, income and quality of genes. Doctors, engineers and military men were his main targets. Military men were always good because of the free perks they got from the government: free car, free telephone, free house, and free servants. Doctors were also preferable although a surgeon was more prestigious. And there was always demand for engineers at home and abroad where salaries could double. Nana spread the word that Boo Boo was looking for a prospective husband.

A young engineer was the first to pay a visit to the house. He was short with a bald head that shone in the candle light. After half a glance Boo Boo disappeared into her bedroom and did not reappear until the man had left and was halfway home in a rickshaw.

'Apart from his breath, what a nice man,' Nana said.

'I'm not marrying him,' was Boo Boo's blunt reply.

'Why not?' Nana seemed genuinely surprised.

'He smells and he's ugly.'

Nana scoffed at Boo Boo's reaction.

'He's an engineer and he has an MSc from Dhaka University.'

'I don't care.'

Nana realised that it wasn't going to be easy persuading Boo Boo to marry. Usually, she listened to her father but when it came to her marriage she wasn't about to fling herself at anyone. As Nana continued to bring in countless eligible young men with round bellies and affluent blood each meeting ended with Boo Boo's blunt rejection.

Nana on the verge of giving up spent nights looking up at the ceiling in total frustration wondering what to do with his pertinacious daughter until he received an enquiry from an eighth suitor and Nana promptly arranged a meeting. Boo Boo caught a glimpse of him standing in the hallway. His skin was the colour of dark chocolate and she lamented to herself 'he's a blacky sambo.'

Nana reminded Boo Boo that, although not the right shade, 'he's in the army and also a doctor. Tall, handsome with very white teeth. He speaks English and writes poetry, what more do you want?'

The promise of being an officer's wife was actually very enticing. Within a month Boo Boo married the doctor and moved to Dhaka. She returned a fortnight later to pick up a few forgotten things arriving in a designer sari with too many gold bangles jangling on her arms. Ripe and radiant, the family crowded around her in slight awe of her transformation. She was unrecognisable. Hidden behind a dazzling burst of purple and gold finery.

Mina didn't find a private moment with Boo Boo and had to share her with Nana. Sitting on the edge of the bed Nana, admiring Boo Boo's glamour, stroked her cheek with his forefinger.

Mina was twenty. She had never kissed a man, never even had a proper conversation with one, never mind anything else.

Boo Boo whispered to Mina "don't worry; they say that if you wear a thread around your belly you'll be married within a week." Boo Boo had already discovered some coarse thread in her sewing bag. Mina passively let her sister tie the thread around her waist but feeling suddenly ridiculous Mina tore it off.

'What is it?' said Boo Boo looking rather bemused.

'Leave me alone.'

'Don't worry, someone will marry you. I mean you'll get somebody eventually.'

'I don't want to get married!' shouted Mina.

'Stop acting like a peasant.'

'I like peasants,' mumbled Mina.

Wrinkling up her nose in disapproval, Boo Boo turned away and unravelled her sari in silence. Unable to sleep, Mina slipped under the bed and, with the clucking of a chicken to keep her company, read her Chemistry book to block out all thoughts of marriage and men.

Mina returned to Dhaka for the solitude of her hostel. With a small plastic bag, and a box of sliced papaya prepared by Nanu, Mina left the house early in the morning escorted to the bus stop by her little brother, Omar. It was a blazing day, not a cloud in the sky. The air was dusty and the leaves on the trees dry and brown, thirsty for a drop. Mina boarded the rickety bus and waved good-bye to her brother. He didn't wave back knowing she'd be home in a week or two. The bus was packed with people until they spilled out the gaps, the air heavy with the odour of sweat and thick with heat. From her window she watched an old man take a leak in a hole made with his big toe. Passing him was a skinny boy with legs covered in swollen welts. He was running and yelling after his friends. As the bus gathered speed the trees melted into a blurred strip and she dozed off. Mina woke up to the sight of scores of people rushing to get off the bus onto a street packed with vendors, young beggars and lounging old men. Jammed with people Mina boarded the ferry and with nowhere to sit she stood by the edge watching the waves batter its' rusty walls. Six hours later, hungry, dirty, and sticky she landed at Shadarghat in Dhaka: a place notorious for muggings and petty crime, a place where shady men skulked in the shadows and stared at the women as they walked by. The light was fading and the water shimmered golden orange. Crows swirled above cawing madly. Mina walked through Dhaka city past the rubbish, the rubble on the streets, the sacks of stuff piled high and through the dust that swirled in great big gusts. She paused to watch a woman taking a bath in the street. The woman poured water from a red bucket over her fully clothed body. Children ran and played by the roadside while others slept rough on the dirt. Hard skin on feet, blackened toes, tattered shorts, skin and bones. There was an on old man; he was half naked, squatting in the middle of the road, with his palm outstretched. A stranger dropped some taka that landed by his feet before walking off. He didn't look him in the eye. 'May Allah be with you,' the old man said quietly. What gave him the will to live? What was his life for? To beg, to sleep, to eat. There were so many like him in Bangladesh and people walked by, apathetic, and hardened by it all. They'd seen it all before. It was nothing new. Mina walked a few steps and saw a kid with stick legs and arms jutting out his body, flies swirled above his face as if he was a corpse, his breathing was heavy, his stomach bloated and his skin black from the beating sun. Two pretty girls in flowery dresses that were two big for their slender limbs sifted through rubbish. The stench made Mina wretch and others keep their distance. How much would these kids make today? What were they looking for in that filth and rot? They sifted with a certain vigour and it made Mina feel sick to watch when one girl clapped her hands because she'd found an old piece of plastic. She walked on as the sun began to sink into the sky through side streets flanked by tiny stores. Scores of rickshaws fought for space down the narrow roads. Mina looked at the buildings in Old Dhaka town, pink and yellow crumble splattered with indecipherable text. Signs, poles, pipes all jutted out like extra limbs. Nothing was smooth and simple. Mina noticed a man sitting quietly watching the world through his small black eyes. He tapped his gnarled toes and his lips were curled in a subtle smile. His beard was long and white like Nana's, his long nose eclipsed his upper lip. He was alone but content and Mina wondered why he looked so calm and peaceful when he had nothing but the clothes on his back. He got up and left down a side street and Mina watched until he disappeared. A lady tossed hot round pittas and the aroma made Mina feel a pang of hunger in her empty belly, but with just enough money to get home she could only savour the warm sweet smell. To the left of the pitta stall sat a young man sewing the sole of a sandal with a needle and thread. He was squatting over a pile of shoes, head bent low, engrossed in what he was doing. The needle moved with a certain grace and alacrity and Mina became slightly mesmerised by the motion. She watched everything and everybody; not wanting to miss anything: the man at his stall rearranging his lychees, the net bulging with live chickens waiting for death, the boy haggling over the price of an egg. She carried on walking to see a crowd of people swell in the street like a stampede of angry ants. Mina saw a man being dragged from a baby taxi, beaten and kicked by a gang of men. The crowd cheered and clapped as another kicked over the taxi and set it alight. The tiny vehicle blew up in flames. The man looked like a terrified small animal, his body was covered in an array of cuts, his face puffy and swollen, his shirt torn, his genitals exposed and he was crying like a child. 'Shut up,' someone shouted and slapped him again. There were no police, just the angry masses intent on killing this man.

'What's going on?' Mina asked one onlooker.

'This bastard tried to rob a passenger, but we got him and now he's in for it.'

'Where are the police?'

'They're bloody useless, we don't need the police.'

'But they're going to kill him.'

'Good, that's what he deserves.'

People continued to jeer every time someone kicked the thief. Each kick and punch felt like a rupture in her belly and Mina had to walk away because she felt pity and revulsion and she didn't know what to do so she escaped into a nearby building and climbed up to the rooftop to get away from the violent babble, the blood, the fumes, the madness. As the sun slipped to bed the bats soared from trees and began to glide overhead flapping their black wings. Where are they going? Mina wondered.

Sanchita Islam

When Mina came down scores of lamps emanating a soft fuzzy glow greeted her. People flanked the narrow dimly lit streets of Dhaka city. A dark faced customer with thick black hair sat with a lungi draped over his shoulders as another shaved his neck delicately. Pictures of women caked in make up and adorned with gold graced the crumbling walls of the barber shop and the customers squinted a little in the green neon light. Mina walked into the night market stall, a suffocating low ceiling boxed off quarter, and started to sweat in the heat. Flies nestled on the corpses of fish, bulbs glowed in the dark and people poked, prodded and haggled. There were baskets, sacks, silver plates laden with thousands of tiny fish, black eyes bulging in the heat, lying in an orgy of death. Mina saw a big Ruee fish and enquired about the price. She had nowhere to cook it in the hostel but she knew that Nana would have bought it. Wiping the droplets of sweat from her brow Mina left the fish market and walked past other stalls and produce. Turquoise bowls spilling with hoards of tiny green chillies, potatoes still encrusted with earth, lumpy carrots, pyramids of leafy vegetables and round hard olives shimmering in the candlelight. She walked on past the bakery; a man inserted a long pole into the burning furnace. Inside the furnace was an array of small dough dumplings that lay on black trays waiting for a roasting. Mina watched the yellow flames, like an angry mouth waiting to eat her. One by one a tiny man shoved in the trays transforming the anaemic gooey dumplings into sweet brown cakes. The smell of dough, yeast and sugar made Mina feel nauseous. How could they work in such a place with no ventilation, no room to move? Another man placed his hand in a huge tin bowl and Mina watched his glistening arms move rhythmically round and round, fighting with the stubborn dough. A thick mattress of white lay on the worktop and another man tore off a small piece. He rolled it into a long rope like structure pinching and squeezing it into a delicate creation. Mina noticed that all the men were half naked and she felt hot in her sari and blouse. Why couldn't she be half naked? Mina walked by a tea stall lined with open cans of condensed milk. A man made tiny cups of sugary tea and a long line of people waited for a taste. The flame from his lamp danced against the wall decorated with red painted Bangla scrawl. He counted the taka and slipped the wad into his top shirt pocket. Mina almost knocked over a bicycle wheel lying in the middle of a crowded street. A man squatted as he twiddled and prodded the wheels. Mina continued to meander through the crowded streets lined with hand painted billboards advertising Nestles milk and antiseptic cream. The lights gave Dhaka city another worldly feel, as if she was visiting a planet inhabited with amorphous beings decorated with light blue neon fuzz. She squeezed by the people, the so many people that seemed to fill every inch of space. They pushed and rushed, she felt small and squashed until she boarded a rickshaw that weaved through the narrow lanes. Mina held onto the sides as her body swayed with the motion, the night air blew her hair in her face and she stretched her head back and closed her eyes. They finally reached Dhaka University town where she escaped into the cool haven of her tiny room at the hostel on Fuller Road.

Several days after Mina left for Dhaka, Nana received a letter from Boo Boo's husband. He mentioned something about a friend of his brother looking for a bride. Should he pass on the details? Nana agreed.

With hair slicked back and wearing a tight suit that lengthened his body a young man arrived at Nana's house accompanied by a woman. They introduced themselves as Ravi and Rina. Nana immediately noted Ravi's fair complexion, his height and the way he said 'hello' in English without an accent.

During the meeting the woman answered for Ravi boasting about his 'top class university education' and his life in Paris and England working in 'finance' She pulled out two sepia tinted photographs from Ravi's pocket and showed them to Nana. In one he stood proudly in Trafalgar Square wearing a broad grin surrounded by flapping pigeons. In the other he strolled through Parisian back streets looking totally at home. Nana stared at the photos examining the buildings, the pigeons and the people in the background with their strange haircuts.

GUNGI BLUES

Rina continued to elaborate on Ravi's plans, 'he's thinking of settling in Bradford. It's a really beautiful place. Just like back home.'

Ravi proudly added 'I'm studying at the Bradford Bank institute to be a Bank Manager.' Nana nodded with approval and the interview was over.

Dazzled by Ravi's looks, his very white teeth, the shine on his shoes and his talk of institutes, Nana gave them permission to see Mina in Dhaka.

For the last few days Mina had spent her life in the library. A dingy place with stale air and baggy eyed students. That afternoon her sari was sticky and face pale from the stress of working on her essay for six solid hours. She found herself hunting for a missing book. It was not on the shelf, not on the trolley; she bent down on her knees and looked under the gap beneath the book-shelf and the floor. At the end of the aisle she saw something hidden in dusty shadow. As she stretched out her arm she felt a gentle tap on her shoulder. Looking up there was a woman and a young man.

'Excuse me, is your name Mina?'

Still kneeling on the floor, Mina nodded feeling quite ridiculous.

'We've come from your father's house.'

Mina's pallor faded and she feared the worst.

'This is my cousin Ravi. I'm Rina.' There was an awkward silence and Rina tried to squash it with a broad smile. 'Your father said that you are studying for your Masters.'

Mina nodded slowly, unsure whether or not to make polite conversation.

'How clever you must be,' said Rina clapping her hands together with exaggerated zeal.

Mina felt wet from a sudden sweat attack. Who were these people? Why had her father sent them? She wasn't supposed to talk to strangers? She should have made an excuse and walked away but she found herself transfixed by Ravi's dimples, his creamy skin and warm smile.

Mina examined them both. Rina was tiny, with nondescript features enhanced with make up and well dressed in a pretty patterned sari of green leaves. Ravi was smartly dressed in a pencil suit, of slim build with a lovely sheen to his hair. They didn't look like suspect strangers; they looked respectable.

There were two rickshaws waiting outside. One of the drivers was sitting in the carriage with his feet balanced on the bicycle seat.

GUNGI BLUES

'Get up,' shrieked Rina, undaunted by the driver's size.

He woke up with a start, almost losing his balance. Rina ignored him and boarded the rickshaw, leaving Mina no choice but to ride with Ravi. It was dusk now and the streets of Dhaka were coming alive with night beggars, burning lamps and street traders. The air was bursting with the sound of honking horns, the whirr of traffic and the clutter of rickshaws. Mina did not say a word to Ravi even though she wanted to. Instead she examined his knee. It looked round and soft. Then she peeped at his shiny black leather shoes. He must have polished them that same morning. And she noticed that his hands were lighter than her hands as if he had always kept them in his pockets to avoid the sun. They travelled into Dhanmondi past Elephant Road where stalls were lit up and masses of people perused the goods. Saris, lungis, punjabis, sandals, ladies shoes, jewellery, handbags and bindis. They sold everything on Elephant Road. 'Would you like anything?' Ravi asked gently. Mina shook her head like a child and looked straight ahead to avoid further temptation.

They soon pulled into the driveway of a medium sized house. It was plain and simple. Rina guided Mina through the hallway into the lounge. There was a single glass cabinet, a small round table, two couches and the floor was bare apart from a patterned red rug.

'Please sit down. Do you want some tea?'

'No thank you,' replied Mina.

Ravi excused himself to the bathroom and left the room and once gone Rina began to talk very fast.

'Ravi's training to be a banker in England and he's going back in a few weeks. We're worried that he might marry an English girl. That would be devastating. That's why we all think it's best you marry as soon as possible.'

Mina's brain froze like the shock of a sudden fall.

'We've already made an appointment at the registry office that's if you want to marry Ravi. The wedding is at midnight, tomorrow.'

Rina paused for a slurp of her tea before saying 'we've sent a telegram to your father but I don't think there will be a problem because he's practically given his consent.'

Seeing the stunned expression on Mina's face Rina softened her voice and said 'you know, just between you and me, when Ravi saw you he whispered to me that he'd fallen in love with you. I swear to Allah that's the total truth.'

GUNGI BLUES

Mina did not recollect any clandestine whispering in ears and became slightly perplexed and excited simultaneously. Ravi re-entered the room and Mina had a good long look. His skin was the colour of coffee cream, his eyebrows straight like two neat hedges, his nose small like hers, his eyes deep set like two small wells, his lips moist from licking and his hair straight with naughty flecks that wouldn't keep in line and fell over his eyes. He didn't resemble the usual men on the street, short and skinny with bad teeth or fat and loud with hairy toes. Mina caught Ravi staring at her again and she felt something inside, the mess of emotion and a quiver like toes playing in hot water.

Rina bombarded Mina with cups of tea and home made sweet things while Ravi wooed her with coquettish looks. Mina could have stayed for hours until she absentmindedly glanced down at her watch and hastily excused herself.

The street lamps glowed feebly as she ran down the street trying to avoid the stares of night strollers. Mina had no idea where she was heading but she continued to run, waving her head like a mad woman to scare away dubious strangers until she heard the tinkle, tinkle of a rickshaw and stepped right into the street to stop it.

The buildings, houses, trees and street all looked unfamiliar to her. She didn't know where she was. After a few minutes the sight of the chipped white gates of the hostel calmed Mina down. She gave the rickshaw driver a generous tip, walked slowly to her room, unlocked the door, sat on her bed and, staring at the wall in the darkness, tried to make sense of the mush in her head. She only saw Ravi's face, his creamy hands and shiny shoes. And in her mind she was in England, living in a little house and lying in bed with him under white sheets. Miles apart from Dhaka, Nana, the tubby neighbour, the man in the Hawaiian shirt and Pathuakali. Marriage seemed like the right thing to do. It was her chance to escape a country where Mina thought women were second class citizens, where women were treated like dirt, born only to serve, obey, cook and have children. She didn't want that life. She wanted to think for herself and use her brain. She lay awake with nothing but the supple fantasies that writhed in her head and wrestled with an aching need to be free.

Nana was walking down the aisles of the market. Squeezing lemons, sniffing coriander, caressing tomatoes. Wrinkled old people squatted by their neatly arranged goods bartering, spitting and chewing. Nana saw a familiar face, a local buying watermelon, with eyes as round as golf balls and a prominent honk of a nose.

'Hello, how are you?' Nana said cheerily.

'So so. What about you and those kids of yours?'

GUNGI BLUES

'I've married off the eldest to a doctor,' Nana said proudly.

'What about the middle one,' the local asked casually.

'She's not married yet but there's been interest.'

'Who from?'

'A chap called Quazi Ravi Islam.'

'Oh I know him,' said the man soberly.

'Do you?' replied Nana excitedly.

'Yeah, I met him in Barisal before he went to London. His mother died when he was ten you know and then his father re-married. The boy had to fend for himself and his seven brothers and sisters. I don't blame him for running off to England like that.'

Nana was bewildered as the local rambled. 'I mean he couldn't afford to finish his studies or anything. And my god you should see where they live. It's in the sticks ... I'll take these three.' He said pointing at several large watermelons.

'How do you know all this?' asked Nana sceptically.

'You know what it's like round here. You can't even fart without someone knowing about it.'

Nana didn't wait to hear anymore and making his excuses squeezed through the crowded market and made his way home. When Nanu saw him empty-handed she asked 'Where's the food?'

Nana's nostrils flared rapidly and like a blast of air he let his fury out on his wife

'Food? Never mind the food. I knew I should have stuck to solid men with solid careers. This Ravi is an uneducated peasant. He has no degree, nothing. He's semi literate. What kind of life can he offer? ... All he can offer is Trafalgar square and shitting pigeons.' He paused before whispering 'She won't do anything without consulting me first will she?'

'You should have checked him out before sending him to Dhaka, you idiot.' Nanu shot back.

'Shut up,' Nana screamed as he clutched his head in exaggerated anguish. He ran to his desk, scribbled down a note and rushed out the house. Running past plodding pedestrians he jumped in a rickshaw.

Nana watched the driver's thin brown legs go round and round, his toes cling onto the pedals and his lungi inflate with air. They were almost there, but an old man crossing the road, carrying sticks on his bent back held up the rickshaw. With each step the old man paused for strength. The driver, along with scores of others, swore and shouted at the old man to hurry up but he ignored them all and took his time. Nana's heart was pounding and he jumped out, running the rest of the way. Wheezing for breath, he glanced at the post office clock. It would close in five minutes and there was a queue of three before him. Nana sighed. The seconds ticked by as the queue barely moved. It was two minutes to five now. The last customer was fumbling with his change. Nana didn't wait for him to leave; he just stuffed the letter under the counter. The man behind the glass had a sallow face with hollow eyes. He flicked through his book and carefully tore out a stamp. Brushing the back of the stamp with water he stuck it on the envelope. Droplets collided with the ink and Nana began to tut and sigh as he watched the ink run. In response the man blew on the envelope and waved it in the air. Nana bit his tongue waiting for him to drop the letter down the shaft.

'Can I send that telegram now?' Asked Nana quickly and he pushed the crumpled piece of paper under the counter. The man screwed up his eyes as he tried to decipher Nana's spidery writing then he proceeded to send the telegram through a series of tick ticks and tock tocks before slowly returning to the counter to his multi coloured stamps. Nana still stood expectantly and watched as the man deliberately ignored him. Nana shouted

'Have you sent the damn thing?' Scowling the man nodded and Nana finally left.

After handing in her final essay, Mina decided to visit the park. A huge place with miles of green grass and tall Deb Daru trees. Families came with their kids. Clandestine lovers held hands behind bushes. Sleeping beggars sought refuge under the shade of leafy branches. Finding a bench to sit on she dreamt of sucking sticks of sugar cane and swimming in the pond at home. The sight of water always made her feel calm. With no water in sight she stared into the matrix of knots and intertwining branches of a tree. It was one big mess and she couldn't tell where one branch ended and the other began.

By two she hurried to the hostel to prepare for her big day, scouring her wardrobe for something to wear. With only two saris to choose from she selected the green one with embroidered peacocks on a red silk boarder. She sat in front of the mirror, resting her head on folded arms and pouted. Her face was scrubbed clean. Fresh but plain. She knew she had some lipstick, an old one she'd stolen from Boo Boo and blunt eyeliner hidden at the bottom of her underwear drawer. Sharpening the eyeliner she drew lines around her eyes and dabbed lipstick here and there. Blending red splodges into luscious lips and rosy cheeks she now looked like a pretty bride. Then she sat and waited for a while. Unable to sit still she looked out the window wondering if they might come early.

GUNGI BLUES

She paced up and down her room desperate to get out. If she left the room, they might come. She stayed put. Tried to sleep. Couldn't sleep. Tried to read. The words flew off the page and slipped away. Then she thought of Ravi. Her future husband. It felt right. Crazy but right. And she began to giggle with excitement and cry with fear. Enormous fluctuations filled her tiny room and she sat swaying in the midst of it all until she heard a loud knock at the door. It was Rina and seeing Mina, she let out an exaggerated gasp 'You look like a Bombay movie star.'

Ravi sat waiting in a white Toyota, wearing a freshly pressed suit and a starch white shirt with a black silk tie. He looked like the fifth member of the Beatles. He chivalrously jumped out to open the car door for Mina and she smiled a smile she'd rather conceal because it exposed everything inside.

The registry office was a grey non-descript building standing in isolation on a street corner. Rina banged on the door with her tiny fists until a tired looking registrar with ruffled hair and moustache guided them into a tiny room with a single light bulb hanging from the ceiling and a large tatty book sitting on the desk in the corner. While flicking out clumps of eye cheese with one hand he introduced himself with the other. Then he straightened out his hair, cleared his throat and began to read the vows. Lasting a mere two minutes Ravi slipped an opal ring on Mina's finger and sealed the moment of marriage with an impromptu kiss that sent a mountain of tingles in her tummy. Signing the book, with a couple of biros, they were officially pronounced man and wife. Congratulating them both with a handshake and a pat on the back the registrar went back to bed saying that 'cheap weddings always make parents happy' and Mina left content. Ravi held Mina's hand in the back of the car and it felt weirdly nice and then they dropped her back at the hostel to spend her wedding night alone.

Mina woke to see sun specks crawling up the wall. As she pottered about her room she sang to herself totally out of tune. A knock interrupted her flow. She opened the door, half-expecting Ravi; it was just a fellow student. 'There's a telegram waiting for you downstairs.' She said.

Mina ran downstairs to the small back office where people sat twiddling pencils and reshuffling papers. An elderly lady with dry hair and a big belly instinctively handed over the telegram and watched with real interest as Mina grabbed it from her hands. Tearing it open she read: 'Mina, a man and a woman are coming to visit you. Stay away from them and do not talk to any strange people.' The telegram was from Nana.

'Anything important?' asked the dry haired woman.

GUNGI BLUES

Mina looked up and replied very calmly 'no' and she crumpled up the paper before passing it to the woman.

Mina watched the dry haired woman throw it and miss the bin by inches. The woman left it on the floor to be kicked around and trampled on. Mina walked back to her room and started to sing again. What could she do? It was too late. She was already married.

Ravi came by to pick her up an hour later, dressed in a navy suit and swirly patterned tie. He greeted Mina with a tight hug and kiss on each cheek that sent tingles in her toes. 'everything is sorted out. Passport, tickets, visa and I've booked a ferry to take us to Barisal for a few days before the flight.' He said happily.

Mina beamed at her new husband, admiring his shiny skin and white teeth but as she went to close the door, she said in a timid voice 'I have to say goodbye to my parents before we go.'

Ravi and Mina took a taxi to the ferry. The sun was dazzling; the air arid, the streets bustling with noise but the hot commotion seemed sublime to Mina and everything looked purple in her eyes. Even the pushing, shoving, poking people didn't fracture her mood.

Finding a tiny corner Ravi took off his jacket before letting Mina sit on the dusty ferry floor.

'Do you want to see my world?' he said not waiting for her reply.

Pulling out a small green book with gold ring binding Ravi handed it to Mina. Tentatively she opened the book and struggling with the thin sheets of tissue, Ravi helped to turn the pages. In the first photo, Ravi leant casually against a wall signposted Kilburn. In the next sat two slender men swaying with laughter. They were young and handsome with good bone structure and Mina couldn't help comparing them with Ravi. Turning the page, Ravi was sitting outside a cafe wearing shades, puffing on a fag. In the distance two chic women, with bouffant hair and wearing pastel coats, walked by grand buildings with intricate facades. Ravi turned the next page and there he stood fighting off dozens of pigeons against a backdrop of strange haircuts and dull clothes. Ravi snoozed on Mina's shoulder as she scrutinised the white women, the handbags, Kilburn station and the red London buses until they became hazy in the fading light.

Landing in Barisal, Ravi saw Mina on to a bus that took her most of the way home. It was packed with people, there were others hanging off the sides, spitting occasionally. A sweaty fat man sat next to Mina squeezing his body close to hers and she remained tense for the rest of the journey. Mina tried to take in the view from her window, the colour of the trees, the tiny shacks for houses, the kids playing by the roadside. She didn't want to ever forget. Dehydrated, dusty and dirty when Mina walked up the mud path she slipped out the back to dip her hot feet in the pond. Nanu was busy in the kitchen, chopping, de-scaling, and scrubbing. Dolu was smoking his coconut pipe in the bush as he wiped mud on a silver pot. Papri was colour co-ordinating her saris. Nana was sitting in his room writing a letter at his desk. Seeing Mina standing in the door way he leapt up and said 'Did you get my telegram?'

Mina nodded and Nana let out a deep sigh.

'Oh thank Allah for that.'

'I'm married,' she said holding up her opal ring.

'What? But I told you to stay away from those people,' he wailed like a wounded animal.

'Yes but it was too late ... don't worry Abu, I'm really happy.'

'Happy.' Nana scoffed. 'Don't you realise he's totally uneducated. He's a peasant compared to you. You could have had brigadiers, generals, doctors, engineers, anyone you wanted.'

Mina watched as Nana began to rant.

'I never said they could talk to you. They were only supposed to look at you, not talk. How dare they talk to you!'

'Rina said she tried to contact you.'

'She never contacted me. She tricked you into marrying that peasant, you idiot.' Nana's anger waned and his voice began to tremble. 'Don't you see, you're like a precious diamond and everyone wants a piece of you.'

'I thought you'd be pleased.' Mina's voice trailed off as she watched Nana break down into sobs and his body collapse into a floppy heap on the bed. His anguish was visible, his tears tangible and Mina's happiness began to fizzle. 'Write to me,' Mina said. Nana didn't reply. There was nothing more to say. Mina slipped away to the kitchen hut and watched Nanu pull the intestines out of the chicken for a minute before entering.

'Do you need anything, any food for your journey?' Nanu asked chopping off a chicken's feet without looking up.

A lump the size of a small coconut swelled up in Mina's throat. 'I'll be fine,' she replied.

'What are you going to do in England?' Nanu said irritably.

'I don't know.'

Nanu quickly resumed her chopping and said abruptly 'have a good journey, look after yourself.' And the conversation was over.

Mina sought out Papri and Dolu. She couldn't find Conna or her brothers. No hug, no kisses just sad eyes. Then Mina walked to the pond at the back of the house and watched the geese snoozing under the leafy shade of the trees, two chickens walked proudly towards her. She looked at the forest thick and lush that went on for miles beyond and fat tears plopped down her cheeks. The light speckled psychedelic patterns on the mud and caressed the water of their tiny pond with a silver kiss. As she walked down the mud path, she didn't look back at the pink house, the house where she was born.

She wanted to be strong but her head was heavy with the sound of Nana's sobs. Heavy with the image of his strung out body on the bed. And when she tried to sleep on the bus, no sleep came, only Nana's words mixed with bumps and jolts.

A rickshaw took her down winding lanes and remote leafy corners. She listened to the sound of noisy crickets and humming wheels in the thick darkness. The rickshaw halted and Mina saw a bright light in a window. Mina asked the driver to stay put and banged on the door. It was open. A burst of voices and laughter invaded the air. Guided by the sounds she entered a crowded room. Ravi leapt up to greet her and all eyes were on her. A chubby man, who faintly resembled Ravi, flapped his arms in excitement at the sight of her. And a tiny girl called Mary stared up at Mina with small beady eyes.

Ravi's other sister Renu was the image of her brother. She watched stealthily from a corner before sitting beside Mina. Making bland small talk she asked 'are you happy then?'

'Yes I am,' replied Mina.

'You just wait,' she said solemnly. 'Everyone's happy at the beginning but it won't last. Things always change.'

'What are you talking about?'

'You'll see,' she whispered.

Mina looked into her face. She had all Ravi's features, eyes, nose and mouth, wide bone structure and well-defined eyebrows but there was something different in her expression and Mina couldn't quite fathom what it was.

Staying up that night Mina enjoyed the fuss and attention. By three o'clock in the morning when Ravi had muttered his last joke people trickled off to bed. With no spare room Mina slept with Ravi's sister polarised at two ends of a small double bed. Mina couldn't sleep. It was thirteen minutes past five in the morning and Mina was lying in a strange and unfamiliar bed in a strange and unfamiliar place. At that precise moment Mina felt utterly alone. She would have liked to run up to the roof and catch the sun waking up but she was scared because there was darkness all around her.

By morning, Mina saw the house in full sunlight, cracks, leaks, mould and all. The house was cramped for six people with no pond in the back and only a small yard in the front. In the wilderness of trees Mina's mind wandered free. She filled her days taking long walks with Ravi, sneaking clandestine pecks in shady spots. In the evenings she watched Ravi animate the room with his talk of Paris and London, and laughed along with the others, even when she didn't get the jokes. On her last day in Barishal she spent it alone in a mustard field by the river. Masses and masses of mustard yellow flowers created a soft bouncy bed for flies and birds to play. A mound of wheat sat on the edge of the field like a swollen carbuncle and Mina watched a woman lead a small goat down a narrow path through the golden field. Her pace was slow, her face weary. In her other hand she carried a bucket full of water. Everyday she fetched water not once, not twice but countless times even though her arms felt heavy and her bones and muscles ached with the pain of it all. Mina got up and walked to the river bank.

A paper pink sun was setting in a red sky as crows flew overhead fighting with swirling cloud tails in a mad rush to get home. The river quietly roared at Mina and she roared back. She was sitting on a pebbled sandy bank under an elegant tree watching a lonely fisherman walk across a grassy green bank to his boat. He was carrying a basket on his tiny head. The sun was low and tickled the peaks of the liquid gold water and Mina imagined that she was at the most beautiful point in the world. She watched as the fisherman climbed into the skinny boat. As he advanced further into the river's mouth Mina shed a tear for him and watched the fisherman diminish into a silver dot. The river ate him up. He wasn't coming home. Mina waited and waited and slowly the skinny fisherman came into view with a net crammed with tiny bony fish that Mina wanted to eat. His skin was totally black, his wide brimmed hat battered and wet, his clothes just a mix of rags. He didn't look sad or happy. His mouth was a thin line that Mina could have drawn with her own hand. And she envied him. She envied his simple existence. She envied his courage to ride the belly of that roaring mass. To ride without fear or contempt.

Mina felt alone again once the fisherman had left. She made patterns in the sand with her finger and realised that if it wasn't for the light and the intoxicating way that it played with the universe she would have given up a long time ago. Perhaps that was what life was about. Light, trees, the sea, the sky and that skinny fisherman. Now her life would be in England with Ravi and Mina had no idea what it would be like, all she knew was there would be no mustard fields, no rivers or fisherman and she felt overwhelmed with a melancholy that was heavy like lead.

A farewell feast was painstakingly prepared on that final day with enough food for thirty people with big appetites. Mary and Renu cried all day and Ravi's brother moped around the house with sagging shoulders.

As they prepared to leave Renu glared at Mina and she watched as the woman's face twisted up as if she'd sucked a whole lemon. Ravi dispelled the difficult moment with a spontaneous embrace. His sister stared into her brother's eyes like an infant school girl with a crush on a junior prefect. Ravi whispered something in her ear and the sharp edge in her eye softened.

After much hugging and crying Ravi and Mina finally boarded the rickshaw. Ravi's brother and sisters stood waving at the rickshaw until it shrank to a colourful speck and there was nothing left to wave at. Looking forward into the trees Ravi was quiet for a while. Then he snapped out of his mood with a slap on his knee. Mina held his hand tight for the rest of the journey until it became sticky like sucked toffee.

When they arrived in Dhaka, Ravi spent the rest of the day with Rina while Mina shut herself away in her hostel. Like a good student Mina sat at her desk and stared down at the page. An hour slipped by. Nothing went in. She eventually found herself rummaging through her sparse wardrobe scouring for shimmering silk saris and the perfect gold ring to stick in her nose. She spent the rest of the day lying on her bed, frowning, pondering, itching her head trying to figure out what to wear, fishing out clothes, making ensembles, trying them on, taking them off, posing in the mirror, making up her face, painting her eyes, desperately trying to look effortlessly beautiful. Finally ready she sat and waited unable to take a nap for fear of disrupting her mascara, unable to do anything apart from wait for that knock at the door. When Ravi arrived and he saw his wife he gazed at her for a moment, admiring her face, her style and understated glamour.

Ravi filled their night with a secret kiss under a tree, creamy ice cream and a Hindi movie bursting with dance, sparkle and a wet sari scene. At the end of the evening they found themselves sitting on a bench in a deserted park. Their elbows touched slightly and their knees occasionally knocked. There was a nippy breeze but Mina felt warm from the quivering hum in her belly as she stared at Ravi's solid, chunky legs, his clean, brown hands and his juicy, pink lips.

Mina beamed and it didn't matter that she'd made Nana cry.

The day came. Mina and Ravi travelled to the airport in a stuffy taxi. The driver kept on itching his balls and gave Mina the dirty eye and when they stopped at a traffic light a girl with a scarred black torso came tapping at the window. Mina was leaving her desh, Bangladesh. Bumpy rickshaw rides, back streets bustling with makeshift market stalls, baby taxis and long rickshaw rides through Gulshan, Banani, Dhanamondi and beyond. People spitting, pissing, hustling, shouting, screaming, sleeping, begging, crying, she would miss it all.

The airport was throbbing and Mina was overcome by scores of staring eyes. She checked her left-hand side. Ravi wasn't there. Trying to sift through the one thousand faces she began to sweat and tremble. She sat down and waited for Ravi to reappear. The sky was a white blazing haze. The trees nestled on the edges like a green fur trim and as Mina sat in the airport she thought of the crumbling walls, the texture of skin on a rickshaw wallah's feet to the dry cake of dirt on a street kid's face. And the light of course. The silver, light that tickled everything it touched. What was there in England? Apart from the freedom to roam without being stared at. How they all stared in Bangladesh? Eyes that pierced Mina and left her wounded, deflated and weak. If only Mina could be invisible and slip through the streets of Dhaka city like water, listen to local conversation, watch the baker knead his dough, the boy frying golden brown pittas, the man weaving his basket by the roadside, deft fingers working like magic. 'If only I could be invisible.' Mina thought. Then she felt a little tug at her sleeve and looking up she saw

Ravi's face loom up like a small full moon. Secure, Mina swallowed her fears in a single gulp and braced herself for a new life in England.

'A midnight marriage,' that's how Mina described it. Ana could imagine her mother doing something impetuous, risking everything for love. She would often talk about escaping from Bangladesh and the suffocating gaze and expectations of family. She wanted to be free. It didn't surprise Ana that her mother had run away to be with a man she hardly knew, to run away to a whole new world. It was crazy. Mad. Ana looked down at the mother, the murmurings continued and she began to talk about the past, about Ravi and Bradford and how it really all began and the stories just flowed out of her like air.

GUNGI BLUES

Brave new Bradford 1968

As Mina prepared to land in London she looked out the plane window and saw a deep blue sky peppered with clouds. Clouds that could have been plucked straight from Pathuakali, but when she squeezed out of the plane the air pinched her toes, the wind seared through her sari and the hairs on her legs stood on end.

'Welcome to Heathrow,' she read. White rectangle blocks, distorted silhouettes and the tail end of planes greeted her as she walked down the plane steps and followed the others onto the bus. With no available seats she stood with her body sandwiched between a sweaty fat man and his skinny fresh-faced wife. Ravi seemed at ease. He lit up a cigarette, flicked away his hair and cut a striking figure in his pencil black suit. He walked on ahead and Mina followed. There were other lost faces, mostly women in saris and open toed sandals, ill prepared for the damp chill of England. They shuffled along, staining the corridors with a spicy odour. Their patterned silk saris, oiled black plaits and mahogany skin clashed with the orange carpet. Reaching passport control, the steady flow came to a halt. A sour mouthed man inspected passports, asked questions and studied faces with uncharacteristic care. Ravi walked through without any hassle. Mina's turn came, she flashed a brilliant smile and said hello politely. The man sitting at the counter didn't smile back, he simply grunted. Scrutinising Mina's passport she waited for the thud of the stamp. It came; she stopped holding her breath and walked past a lady with stiff lacquered hair. She was a big lady, with droopy tits and wobbly arms, multiple frowns and sallow skin. She stared at Mina, long and hard. Mina tried to slip past her but the big lady grabbed her arm. She didn't ask, she just said

'Come with me please?'

Feeling the rapid sear of panic under her skin she looked for Ravi. Too deep in the crowd she only saw a mass of heads all squished together into one. The big lady escorted Mina down an empty corridor and opening a side door pushed Mina into a dingy back room. The door closed behind her and in her pure white sari Mina almost glowed against the dark interior. An old man, wearing a cheap navy suit and a watery smile, sat behind a makeshift desk. Eyeing her up, the old man asked bluntly.

'Do you speak English?'

Mina nodded.

Walking over to the sink by the far wall the old man lathered his hands into thick white foam, before rinsing them three times. Carefully drying his hands on a green paper towel he said 'the reason why you've been brought here is for a medical examination. Do you understand?'

GUNGI BLUES

He stared at Mina, waiting for some kind of response but she just stayed mute.

'I assume, by your silence, that you understand. We don't have much time so could you get undressed now?' he said slowly and loudly.

'What?' said Mina half-scoffing.

The old man stared at Mina. 'Look, we have to check each and every one of you. God knows what you people might bring over,' he said raising his voice.

'Well I haven't brought anything over,' said Mina.

Growing impatient the old man advanced towards Mina and reaching for her shoulder muttered 'I don't have time for this. Take off your blouse or you'll be on the first plane back to where you belong.'

The old man watched as Mina's fingers slowly unbuttoned her blouse.

'Your bra please,' said the old man getting off on Mina's fear.

Unhooking her bra two plump breasts fell out of their hard cups. Keeping her eyes fixed to a dirty patch on the floor she felt the hard skin of his palms and the pinch of his nails. He prodded, poked and squeezed. And she watched him skulk around her naked torso until he returned to his desk to scribble something in a tatty book.

Mina hastily tried to put on her bra but in her struggle with fiddly hooks and stringy loops she took twice as long. The old man walked up to her, not waiting for her to finish and shone a light in her face.

'Now open your mouth wide.'

'Open your eyes,' he continued.

'Look straight at me.' Mina looked reluctantly into his face, observing his lined skin, the red veins clustered round his nostrils, his wet lips and crooked teeth.

'Can you raise your head and keep it there?' He said impatiently and, holding her soft cheeks in his rough hands, he adjusted her head like a plastic doll.

'That's better' he said flashing the light into her eyes just long enough to make her squint.

'Let me just check for lice,' he said pushing down her head with all the care of a builder. Then he scraped her scalp with a metal comb and examined it carefully in the light.

After a minute he said 'you can go now.' Then he walked to the sink and washed his hands with a block of white soap.

With her sari hanging from her shoulders, her hair in a messy heap and tears waiting to spill, Mina rushed out. Half running down the corridor she saw the big lady escorting a young girl. The girl must have only been sixteen; her hair was bound in two plaits, her face round, her skin soft, and her eyes wide. The big lady smiled at her but Mina didn't smile back. Instead she walked on ahead, avoiding the stares of uniformed figures. Mina followed the other women in saris and as she travelled down an escalator she saw scores of people shouting at one another in Bangla, fighting over trolleys, wrestling for space. She saw bodies stacked up against the conveyor belt and anxious faces waiting. Waiting for battered black cases, boxes tied up in string and caskets stuffed with homemade chutney. Standing far from the babbling crowd, Ravi puffed deeply on a cigarette. He cut a striking profile in his black suit and slicked back hair with strands that flopped, James Dean style, over his forehead. Glancing up he saw the white figure of Mina running towards him.

'What is it?' asked Ravi softly when he saw his wife's eyes swell.

'I was examined by this doctor. It was awful. I wouldn't treat a dog like that.'

'What happened?' demanded Ravi.

'I don't want to talk about it' replied Mina unable to control her trembling lips.

She tried to re-compose herself but the quiver in her lip wouldn't stop and the tears oozed out faster than she could wipe them away. Onlookers stared. Seeing a woman cry provided welcome relief from the chaos of the airport. Keeping her head down and letting her hair fall in front of her face Mina's face creased up into a myriad of wrinkles and tears dug slender rivers in the soft ground of her cheeks. Ravi watched silently on as his wife tried to gulp down the emotion swelling like a melon in her throat. It only lasted a few minutes. Wiping the wet snot from her upper lip with a sari end, Mina took a deep breath and looked out at the creaking conveyor belt. She was annoyed that she had cried in public, that people had seen her sniffling, that Ravi had seen her broken and fragile. She straightened up, tried to act like nothing had happened. Her eyes were wide, a little blood shot and her lips were clamped shut. Words fought inside desperate to hurl foul insults at that old man. But there was no time for that. There was no time to reflect only move through the thick of the crowd and wait for the luggage and if she concentrated hard enough that old man might disappear. But he was still there. Poking around in the back of her subconscious with the other two.

GUNGI BLUES

For Mina the sum total of her possessions were packed into one puny case and her heart skipped a beat when she saw it appear squashed under another. Ravi had at least two suitcases and a succession of smaller bags. There was nothing left in Barisal. Grabbing their stuff, Ravi and Mina speeded towards the exit. One dewy-eyed woman, dressed in open toed sandals and a cotton green sari, stared at the emptied contents of her suitcase piled high on a metal counter at customs control. A uniformed man was sieving through the contents. His burly colleague was sniffing at a jar of home made something, dissecting a lovingly wrapped package and poking at another. Mina could smell another nasty trauma brewing; she looked away and rushed on ahead. When she turned round the corner she saw scores of people holding up flimsy cards with names written in felt tip. There was no one in the crowd waiting for them. No long distant relatives. No good friends. No chauffeur to drive them to Bradford. They ended up queuing up behind twenty shivering bodies for a black cab.

Mina listened. Listened for the tinkle tinkle of rickshaws, the fierce crowds and side street vendors. All she heard was the clash of metal, the rumble of cars and low chatter. Looking up her first vision of London was grey pavement slabs, grey roads and grey looking folk pushing trolleys.

'Yes luv,' said the cab driver to Mina. She looked blank and Ravi swiftly intervened with 'Victoria, please.'

Ravi and Mina finally left the fluorescent glare of Heathrow. They didn't say much to one another in the cab. Ravi was too busy counting the luggage, searching his trouser pockets and sifting through old scraps of paper. Mina looked out the window and saw the grey concrete of the road. Her eyes drifted up to the sky. Overcrowded with clouds, plump and heavy. There was a grey sheen to the air. Within minutes she heard the steady pit pat plop of rain against her cab window, transforming her view into a blurred smudge of cars and grey. After forty minutes the rain stopped, a slice of light cracked through the grey and Mina looked out to see tall, narrow London houses lining the road and a burst of pink cherry blossom from a single tree. They turned a corner to see concrete splendour, men in suits, blokes in ill fitting black Macs, women in bright coats and the big hair she'd glimpsed in Ravi's photos. She saw a couple holding hands, flapping flares, long lank hair and an Afro. Flower boxes. Intricate facades. Crumbling brick walls. Shiny wet streets. White stone buildings three storeys high. Dazzling, shop fronts. Red buses. Black cabs. Rushing people. Flapping pigeons. And Mina stared.

The cab turned into Victoria station. It was mad with people. Mad with people queuing for tickets, people sprawled out on seats, people running for coaches, people in need of assistance. Mina stuck close to Ravi and he swiftly guided her through the mess of people onto a coach filled with saggy skin and wrinkles. She observed an old man, sitting adjacent to her. He had small ears, beardy face, tufty white hair and slept with his mouth open. The woman squashed beside him had a triple chin that ate into her neck, a face like a gerbil and wiry hair streaky with white. She wore gold-rimmed glasses, pearls, saggy tights and brown lace up shoes that bulged with crooked toes. Nasal chatter clogged up the silence and the words glazed over her as she stared out the coach window. There was an absence of light, which gave everything a dull hue. And as the coach rumbled out the city and the road branched into the motorway, Mina saw nondescript slithers of bush and concrete, followed by slices of green, the odd munching sheep, funny looking trees and the smoking chimneys of tiny houses dotted over vast fields that stretched for miles. Fields filled with nothing much apart from the occasional cow. Strange looking cows, weighed down with bloated bellies; fat and pasty. Triple the size of the cows in Pathuakali. The fields gradually blended into hills; great big undulating hills. Hills that Mina wanted to climb to the very peak, shout, dance, jump up and down and then take a snooze in the rain. Mina suddenly felt excited. Excited by the lush hills, the fluffy clouds in the sky and the plump cows bingeing on grass. Excited by what she'd tasted in London: the towering buildings, the chiselled facades, the flash cars, the insane rush and the pink of the cherry blossom. Somehow the smell of stale pee emanating from the two crusties in the coach didn't dampen her spirits. She just held her breath, clenched her fists and longed for brave new Bradford.

GUNGI BLUES

First Glimpse

Mina looked out and saw grassy plains, purple patches of heather and black stonewalls worming over green stretches. The whole sky, crowded with heavy black clouds dissected with threads of light, seemed intent on squashing the little people down below. The coach rumbled on through narrower streets and Mina observed the tiny shops, the low houses and the black tiled rooftops. It was small. Up and down. Higgledy-piggledy. After ten minutes they seemed to be entering the town centre. Mina saw a red brick Odeon cinema sat next to the Alhambra Theatre with funny looking portholes lining the front and at the bottom of the road was a massive Morrisons supermarket. There were smaller shops dotting the streets but the Odeon and Alhambra were the focal point of the city. Huge and imposing they gave Bradford a certain presence. Mina imagined that flash things went on in those buildings. They made her feel she was arriving at an important place.

The coach turned down a few winding roads until they entered the station cluttered with fleets of grimy coaches. There was a familiar pushing, shoving and tutting as people elbowed one another in the struggle to be the first to leave. Ravi and Mina waited their turn and ended up the last to get off. Dragging cases, boxes, knotted plastic bags and things tied up in string, they stood at the back of a long winding taxi queue. She looked back at the coach station with its stone floor and bare walls.

The place was filled with sluggish lumps of old people staggering with their bags, in need of assistance but not getting any. With faces lined and weathered, watery eyes, varicose veins travelling up the backs of legs, lacquered white curls, shiny baldheads and hairy ear lobes. Mina looked away and as she stood in line she listened to the whinges and gripes of the gummy man and saggy tights woman standing in front of them. Each word was smothered in a thick accent. Words that mutated into truncated sounds and sharp grunts. Looking disconcerted, Mina didn't understand a word.

After a five minute cab ride they reached a long row of nondescript houses with paved front gardens, black bin bags dumped on kerbs, a dog tied to a lamp post and a kid chucking stones down the drain. When Ravi rang the doorbell a tiny old lady wearing black ankle socks and pink fluffy slippers with thinning strawberry grey hair opened the door. On seeing Ravi her thin-pursed mouth let out a cry of delight and grabbing him by the neck she planted a wet kiss on his chin. The lady's name was Ellie.

Ellie took their coats and hung them on the banister with some difficulty. Ravi tried to help but Ellie wasn't having it. Mina noticed the patterned wine carpet, worn down to the weave in places. She noticed the chipped skirting board; the brown smears on the wall, the narrow hallway, the low ceilings, and the single light bulb smothered in a web of dust and dead flies.

GUNGI BLUES

As soon as she saw her, Ellie stretched out a bony hand and pulled Mina out with a sharp tug.

'Ooh is this your wife? Don't you two make a pretty picture?' she gushed looking Mina up and down. Mina looked angelic, all in white. The brown of her skin glowed against the stark backdrop of silk. The only make up on her face was the shiny blood red of her lipstick.

'Haven't you got lovely lookin' feet?' exclaimed Ellie staring at Mina's elegant long toes.

'Thank you' replied Mina not fully understanding the compliment.

'I'm not showin' you mine with me bunions and corns,' laughed Ellie.

Mina noticed how Ellie's face was ravaged with lines, her eyes sunken, her lips two slithers of pink but you could see a twinkle in her watery blue eyes and warmth in her gummy smile. And there was something endearing about the clumps of mascara in her lashes and the silver blue eye shadow applied to one lid only.

'Are you sure it's all right we stay the night. You see our flat won't be ready until tomorrow' asked Ravi changing the subject.

'Oh shut up, of course it is,' insisted Ellie.

Ellie began to climb up the stairs with a slight limp and a wheeze apologising, every other minute, for being so slow. She heaved as she reached the top of the stairs. And with a shaky hand she turned the door handle. The room was tiny; the size of Dolu's sleeping hut. The wallpaper was peeling and the floor bare with wooden splintered boards. There was a musty old smell that Ellie tried to mask with Rose fragranced air freshener. The light was dim apart from a chink of light that escaped through the curtains. There were flower-patterned curtains, frilly edges on the bedspread and a withering Daffodil placed in a milk bottle on the bedside table.

Ellie walked up to the bed and smoothed out a minuscule wrinkle. Pausing over the bed, she plumped up a sagging pillow. Ravi patted her veiny hand and placing his arm around her fleshy waist, escorted her across the landing to her room. Ravi opened her bedroom door. A mass of clothes lay on the floor, the bed was unmade and curtains drawn. Ravi pretended not to see anything and smiled as Ellie waved goodnight. Then he returned to Mina and lay on the bed. From his perch he watched Mina mess with her bag and blow her nose. Although Mina kept her back to Ravi, she could feel his eyes on her as she looked out the window.

Facing her were rows upon rows of tiny houses with funny looking chimneys, luminous windows, shifting silhouettes and net curtains. Ash clouds and splinters of blue night-light lit up the sky. Curvy hills and tiny trees that looked like flimsy paper cut outs lined the horizon. She looked at the houses with their bricked up back yards, the washing hanging from the lines, the fenced up walls, and the absence of green bush. It was eerily quiet. No crickets, no cawing of crows, just the faint sound of the odd passing car.

Bradford was a brown, black and grey world; so different from the rich green and dusty light of Pathuakali. Momentarily Mina felt a pang in her stomach, could have been hunger, but it felt like sadness and excitement and fear and yearning all at once. Bangladesh was now an abstract distant place. Everything that had been familiar was now remote. A new life was beginning with Ravi and she had no idea how she should behave or what she should say.

Mina stood still now. After a minute she heard Ravi's footsteps creep up behind her. Her body tensed up. Felt his hand squeezing her shoulder and his unravelling fingers. Falling silk by her feet followed swiftly by the blouse. Mina stood in ill-fitting cotton undies, feet hidden under crumpled silk. Ravi looked her up and down. Feeling all shy she placed her hands in front of her body to conceal those tempting bits of flesh. Ravi removed her hands, pulled down her panties and unclipped her bra. She now stood naked before him and when Ravi looked at her body he saw soft flesh and round breasts like two ripe mangoes. Nipples like brown buttons. Long fingers and elegant toes. Legs downy with hair that had never been shaved. Shoulders round and smooth. Holding her trembling hand he guided Mina to the bed. It was barely big enough for two. As Mina lay down she felt a spring jut into her shoulder and when she turned the bed squeaked. Ravi wrapped his arms around Mina slipping his fingers over her soft marshmallow breasts. Cupping the heavy flesh he squeezed it tight. Awkward and scared Mina froze. She'd never lain in bed naked. Her night dress had always formed a protective barrier between skin and sheets. Ravi's fingers were all over her like eager ants. And when he touched her skin a quivering whoosh surged through her body, like the rise and fall of travelling over a sudden bump, but her body remained taut like stretched elastic. Perhaps it was because they were in Ellie's house, lying in a bed where others had slept. Perhaps it was the creaks and lumpy springs. Or perhaps it was because she barely knew the man lying naked beside her.

Ravi looked Mina in the eye and kissed her full on the mouth. Their teeth clashed. She felt the soft gooiness of gums and tongue, all tingly and wet. In the dim light and squeaks Ravi heaved his body on top of Mina. His cock was hard and he tried to ram it between her thighs but she squeezed her legs tight and pushed him away.

Ravi rolled over reluctantly but during the night Mina felt his body pressed close to hers, so close their skin stuck together with the glue of their sweat. Ravi's hand firmly gripped her breasts and she felt his prickly balls press against her. Mina began to stroke his thigh with her little finger. How smooth and soft it was, like the finest silk sari skin, much softer than her skin. Her fingers then drifted down his leg and Ravi whimpered in pleasure. Mina pulled Ravi's hand from her bosom and held it tight but his fingers returned to the security of her breast. She liked the warmth from his palm, the firmness of his grip. He rolled over and Mina stared at the back of his head. His hair was slightly thinning. Mina became worried that Ravi might become a baldy; she carefully re-arranged his hair and it calmed her down a little. And as she lay there stroking his hair she thought how only yesterday she was in Dhaka reading books in sweltering heat, looking for Chemistry books in the library, attending lectures and thinking of PhDs; now she was in Bradford, sleeping naked beside her husband. She missed home, her parents and first light. She'd given it all up for this strange country. And she felt bad because she'd escaped to be free.

First Morning

Ravi was already dressed looking fresh and polished standing next to their bags zipped, knotted, padlocked and ready to go. Mina slid under the duvet, trying to hide her birds nest hair do, crusty eyes, puffy cheeks and snuggled deep in the darkness. Felt safe and warm. It felt like she was back under her bed in Pathuakali but she wasn't. She was in a hard bed in Bradford. Mina's toes wiggled uncontrollably. That's what her toes did when she was nervous. And she was. Nervous to be alone with this man in her weird new world.

Ellie was singing mindlessly as she arranged a damp tea towel by the kitchen sink. Her kitchen was plain with white cupboards that had turned a shade of grey and a matching white floor that was pleading for a mop. A yellow tablecloth brightened up the interior but the place smacked of neglect and old. There were cracks in the wall, a speckle of mould along the sink and a cluster of cobwebs in one corner. She struggled with a pair of Marigold gloves, cursing at them, as her thumb slipped into the wrong finger hole. She searched the soapy depths of her sink and produced a plate. It was covered in egg that had been left there to harden for days. Using a teaspoon she tried to scrape off the yellow gunk. She gave up after two seconds and picked up a mug instead. It was stained brown from strong tea. Despite vigorous scrubbing with her J-cloth, the brown refused to shift. She looked at the pile of dishes, half-empty cups and two greasy frying pans that had been waiting a week for a drink of washing up liquid. Hearing Ravi's footsteps enter the kitchen Ellie impetuously swept the whole lot in the sink.

Ravi saw two pieces of burnt toast sitting on yellow plates. An open jam jar streaky with margarine, an empty tub of Flora and two runny eggs wobbling in transparent jelly. While he munched on his toast, Ravi noticed the hole in the tablecloth, the brown lino that used to be white, the battered cupboards and the light bulb dressed in thick cobwebs.

'How's your egg?' Ellie asked anxiously.

'Perfect,' Ravi replied with his mouth full.

Mina appeared in the doorway dolled up in a bright red sari with lipstick to match looking slightly overdressed for runny egg and burnt toast. She stared at the drab interior, the dirt, the mess, the dishes spilling out the sink. The unfamiliar smell of old fat and fried egg clogged up the air and Mina felt like going back to bed but the old beaming lady made her stay.

Mina looked down at her plate. Where was the moruba fruit and home made yoghurt? She stared at her egg swimming in oil. The smell of oil, egg and toast made her feel sick. She took a sip of her orange juice; it was too sweet so she added some salt. Ravi gave her a funny look. Mina didn't think she was doing anything wrong. She tried a piece of toast and seeing Mina struggling to eat Ravi gently said 'Ellie, we really have to go now.'

Ellie guided them to the front door and watched them put on their coats. Unable to control the emotions churning insider her, she flung her arms around Ravi's neck, squeezing it tight with the affection of a mother saying good-bye to her son. Not to exclude Mina she smacked a wet kiss on her cheek.

Walking down the path weighed down by bags Mina paused to look back at Ellie's house. The pipes and ledges were in need of fresh paint, the windows dying for a scrub, the hedgerow a chop. Ellie stood in her doorway watching them shrink into two specks. When they disappeared round the corner she went back inside.

Mina dragged her feet along the street, pausing every five minutes for breath. The cheap plastic handles ate into her hands, pinching her skin pink. As she stumbled along Mina thought of back home where she would have simply got Dolu to help or climbed into a rickshaw, where she would have travelled in style, shading her face from the glare of the sun. Where she would have sat back and relaxed, watching the passers-by, the kids with their home made toys, the women with baskets poised elegantly on heads and the beggars with their bundles tied heavily with string. Mina's face was dripping with sweat, strands of hair stuck to her face, her lips were chapped, her mouth dry. She wanted to sit under the cool shade of a tree but there was nowhere to sit. In the distance she saw the faint green of hills and the promise of something. But when she looked down the street, the houses looked the same and went on forever. There were hardly any people; the air was heavy with stale smells and the light bland like dull skin.

Ravi entered the Newsagents. It was sandwiched discreetly between two houses. There was a hand painted sign outside the glass front. It read POPS NEWSAGENTS. Pops was long and narrow with a cracked lino floor decorated with a pattern of dirty footprints. The air reeked of stale spice, cigarette smoke, cheap perfume and dogs. At the front of the shop was an array of vegetables: aubergines, shrivelled green chillies and tomatoes that were growing squishy and wrinkly in their plastic crates. Along the sides Mina saw the glossy cover of Vogue and the bold print of the newspapers. Mina stared at the pouting blond on the cover and feeling suddenly inadequate she turned away. Stacked high in the corner were boxes of Salt 'n Vinegar Walkers crisps and at the front of the counter were neatly arranged Rowntree Fruit Gums and green packets of Wrigley's chewing gum. Cutting through the centre of the shop were shelves crammed with Jacob's crackers, McVities digestive biscuits, cock-a-leekie soup, canned carrots, HP brown sauce and Ambrosia rice pudding. An 'Off Licence' sign written in childish hand hung above a vast array of cheap wine and spirits. Mina surveyed the interior with its worn fittings, its Mr Kipling jam tarts and Curly Wurlys. And she wondered what was a jam tart and cock-a-leekie soup? Behind the shop counter stood a round-faced lady wearing a thick red jumper under a beige sari with two large blusher spots gracing each cheek. With her small set eyes and hook of a nose, she was busily serving a customer in a thick accent.

'Can an' Bottle.' the woman said to a man wearing a Mac and clumpy boots.

'Yer what luv,' replied the man checking his pocket for pennies.

'Can an' bottle,' she repeated calmly.

'Can an' bottle. What are yer on about luv?'

'Can an' bottle?' she repeated impatiently.

The man looked bewildered. Before he could utter a response she shot out from behind the counter and started screaming at a scrawny schoolboy in the corner:

'You pucker, you mother pucker. Put my Hula Hoops back you pucker.'

She pulled out the packet from under the boy's baggy jumper, practically crushing it in her fist, and yelled:

'Now puck off you pucker.' The boy ran out the shop and didn't look back. Mina watched on knowing that the boy had stuck something else down his shorts. When she returned to her counter, the man had selected a bottle of Holstein Pils.

'You want bottle,' said the woman itching her armpit before thrusting the bottle into the man's palm. With lightning speed she took his money, cashed it, gave him his change and nodded at Ravi and Mina.

'Yes please luv,' said the woman impatiently.

Mina noticed the bulge of her stomach poking out under her cardigan. Her make up was heavily applied, her blusher too red, her perfume too strong. There was a side door by the counter that led to a back room where the telly was on. Mina saw the back of a turban half concealed in a film of cigarette smoke and a hand resting limply by an ashtray. The man seemed oblivious to the clash of the till and the 'forty pence please.' He was too engrossed with the Snooker.

'Packet of Silk Cut,' said Ravi trying to gage eye contact with the woman.

The woman heaved a great big sigh and looking Ravi straight in the eye, shouted 'which Silk Cut you want?' Pointing at the multitude of cigarettes stacked up behind her.

Ravi silently pointed the packet out and when her back was turned he pulled a face. Mina smirked and the woman whipped round to give them both a dirty look. A look that made Mina feel rather small.

'Do you sell deodorant as well?' Ravi asked.

'Over there.' The lady pointed to shelf stacked with Mum deodorant and Ravi gestured Mina to get one.

A short queue had built up of two old ladies pulling shopping trolleys and a man in a cloth cap. And the musty odour of old mingled with the spicy perfumed cigarette air.

'Next please ... twelve and a half pence please ... Yes please luv ... twenty six pence please,' barked the woman.

Mina watched with a certain fascination, as the woman threw change into palms, tutted with impatience and slammed her till shut before Ravi tugged at her sari to leave. How rude, Mina thought. There was no need to throw money at people. No need to treat them like animals.

Ravi handed Mina the deodorant and said 'this is for you.'

'What for?' asked Mina.

'You need it, you smell,' said Ravi walking on ahead.

Mina washed everyday. She always considered herself clean. Bruised by Ravi's remarks, they walked up the main road in silence. They passed semi-detached houses furnished with potted plants in the windows. Past little side streets called Drummonds, Darfield and Holfield. Holfield was just off Tree Lane. Looming tall and proud was an old church, built with ancient blocks of black stone. And as they turned into Holfield Road, Mina saw the stark backdrop of Bradford. A multitude of rooftops and tiny stone houses stretching far and beyond; reminiscent of Dhaka with its white rickety structures and uneven lines. She saw rubbish on the pavement and weeds sticking through the cracks. The houses were painted in greying shades of peach and white with pillars marking each door. Mina admired the delicate cherub figures carved in the stone pillars; she ignored the chips in the walls. Without the sign stuck in the window, 13 Holfield Road simply looked like another house on a street of houses, not a bank.

'It's a Manor house,' said Ravi rather proudly, 'look at the pillars'.

Mina liked the idea of living in a Manor House. It sounded rather grand, no one needed to know about the litter and the dog shit.

Ravi pushed the door open and walked inside to find no customers, only a skinny man reading a newspaper under his desk. Ravi tapped on the glass window with a two pence piece and the man looked up to see Ravi's smiling face. Ravi introduced himself in Bangla and fifteen minutes later the man emerged with a set of keys. He pointed to a narrow flight of stairs that led to a tiny landing and three rooms. A kitchen, bathroom and a third room that was shut. Ravi opened the door with the key. The room was plain apart from the daisy-patterned wallpaper. The furniture was a mis-match with an overdose of brown to match the worn carpet. There was no duvet on the small bed only yellowing sheets. And the living room consisted of two chairs shoved next to the bed. Dingy and dark Mina opened the greying net curtains, hoping for some kind of view. She saw a grocer's shop at the far end of the road and a tiny bookshop with a sparse display in the window. And there was a woman dumping a shopping bag on the street. She wore a pink cardigan tucked into her sari with thick green socks that poked out her skimpy sandals.

Mina looked around, half-dazed. Sitting on the edge of the bed she took deep breaths while Ravi bustled around unpacking and rearranging the furniture.

Mina stared at the bed. Half falling apart with chipped headboard and stained pillows; the dirty floor looked more enticing. She lay down on the lumpy mattress and with every turn Nana's cries filled her head. She saw Nana weeping on the bed. She saw the pond where she used to swim every day. She saw her brothers and sisters. Mina remembered that there were no hugs or kisses from Nana or Nanu. At the time she didn't mind because she was too drunk on her adventure, too inflated with love for Ravi, too excited by her new life and new freedom. No one could tell her what to do in her life, she could do whatever she wanted. She was so lucky. Luckier than the women she'd left behind who had no lives, no voices, no rights. Women back home were born to serve and be battered like her mother. And she felt pangs of guilt that she'd escaped to pursue her happiness.

Later that afternoon Mina woke up to find Ravi had gone out. She got up and started to potter about the room trying to make it look nice. She saw their cases heaped in the corner and started to unpack Ravi's suitcase. She discovered carefully matched socks, neatly folded ties and perfectly pressed shirts. There was something concealed in a towel. It was a green photo album with gold binding, similar to the one Ravi had shown her on the ferry. Curious Mina opened it. There was a photograph of Ellie standing in front of her semi, wearing familiar black ankle socks and slippers. Her mouth was open in mid laughter exposing three teeth. In the next photo Ravi was sitting on a bench flanked by two white women in mini skirts boasting pointy breasts. Ravi looked totally at home with his legs wide apart and his arms around both girls. Mina noticed Ravi's happy face, his bright eyes and deep dimples. And she examined the thin lips, strange hair, narrow eyes, yellow teeth and round fleshy knees of the woman sitting next to him. Mina closed the album and returned to Ravi's socks. He walked in carrying milk and eggs.

'Who are those women in your album?' Mina asked coolly.

'Which women?' Mina opened the album and pointed at the picture.

'That's Dimna and her friend,' Ravi said awkwardly.

'Dimna, what a funny name' said Mina.

'Dimna's a lovely name. It's very unusual.'

'Who is she then?'

Ravi took a deep breath and his face turned sullen

'She was my girlfriend before I met you,' said Ravi slowly.

Mina felt a strange sensation in the pit of her stomach, as if someone had tampered violently with her internals. Ravi, not waiting for a response, continued,

'I wanted to marry her. You see, I was in love with Dimna.' His voice began to shake thinking perhaps he'd said too much but now he'd started he couldn't really stop. 'I've always liked English girls. They are not that different from Bangladeshi women. I have a very good friend. He married an English lady and she cooks fish so well you wouldn't believe it.' His voice drifted off and he shifted to the window.

'Have you seen that? I never noticed it before. There's a bookshop just opposite us.'

Ravi pressed his face against the window until his nose was squished flat.

Mina didn't respond. She was too busy watching her finger aimlessly follow the contours of the flower pattern on the bed spread in numb disbelief that Ravi was telling her all this now.

Ravi grew quiet, as if waiting to be probed, and Mina reluctantly obliged.

'When did you meet her then?'

'Who?' said Ravi trying to act casual.

Mina's fingers began to pick at stray threads and she hesitated before saying
'Dimna, of course.'

There was a faint strain of emotion in Mina's voice but Ravi didn't turn round. He started to talk fast.

'We met a year ago in London. I was a junior at a bank and Dimna worked there too. I remember when I first saw her. She was standing behind me wearing this pink dress. She was wearing kitten heels, no tights because it was too hot and her dress seemed to stick to her body. I couldn't help noticing her. Anyway, I just introduced myself and that's how it all started really.'

Mina was laying on the bed with her back to Ravi. Part of her didn't want to hear anymore but despite herself she stayed quiet and listened.

'We started to go for drinks at the local pub after work. It became a habit. Sometimes I didn't even have to ask. We'd get funny looks in the pub, mostly from white men. I think they thought I'd kidnapped her. It was complicated with me being Bangladeshi but I couldn't help it, I had to see her. There was a lot of sneaking around behind her parents' back. It was stupid, I mean we were adults but we still played it safe. Usually we ended up sitting on a park bench kissing like teenagers until the attendant threw us out.'

Ravi's body grew animated with the memories but he still didn't turn to face his wife.

'I proposed to her after work in the park. It wasn't planned, it just came out and I couldn't believe it when she said yes.'

Ravi started to sift through his socks and ties as he talked 'I'd never met her parents and Dimna wanted their approval so I had to meet them, even though I didn't want to. I was worried that they wouldn't accept me.'

GUNGI BLUES

Ravi put down the socks and sat on the edge of the bed. He was looking down at his shoes in concentration.

'When I got to her house I wore my best suit and I brought white lilies for her mother. Cost me a fortune but I was trying to be a real English gentleman. I was so sick with nerves. I rang the doorbell, and Dimna's father opened the door. He was bald and stocky. His shirt wasn't ironed and his trousers were too big. I thought he looked a little eccentric but his eyes were cold; he didn't shake my hand he just muttered at me to come in. Then they kept me waiting in the kitchen for half an hour. I was left sitting listening to the dripping tap. I caught glimpses of Dimna's mother skirting around in their neat hallway with its fluffy maroon carpet and perfect white walls. She never once came in, never even offered me a cup of tea. She was a fat version of Dimna.'

Ravi got up to stand by the window and he wished that he'd hidden the album in a better place.

'I was left alone for twenty minutes. Then I heard Dimna rowing with her father in loud whispers. 'Over my dead body are you marrying that half educated Paki.' Dimna argued back and said 'he's not a Paki, he's training to be a bank manager, he's well travelled, he's been to Paris and everything.' Dimna's father just didn't want to know. He couldn't be bothered to talk to me. In the end Dimna walked in.'

Ravi’s voice trailed off but he forced the words out. Mina’s eyes were still closed as she listened. The words were going in her head but her brain was dormant, refusing to register what was being said.

‘She’d been crying. Her eyes were all blood shot and I wanted to tell her parents to go to hell but I knew there was no point. Dimna wouldn’t leave her family for me. We never officially broke it off but we didn’t have to. I never heard from her again. I was devastated and broke down. I couldn’t stop crying. You can't imagine the pain I went through. I didn’t try and call her because I knew it was a waste of time. I decided to get out of England. I needed to clear my head so I went back home to Dhaka and that’s when I met you. It’s funny.'

'What's so funny?' said Mina stonily.

'Funny the way things turn. I was so very fond of English girls and I ended up with you.' Ravi laughed and glanced back to see Mina’s twisted body, her creased up legs, her bent back, and her stiff neck. He walked over to the bed and put his arm on Mina’s waist. The hand felt heavy, like a lead pan. Mina didn’t want that hand anywhere near her but she let it stay. There was numbness spreading through her body like a thick glue that left her stuck.

Mina’s dream was shattered. But if she was honest she didn’t really know what that dream was. A dream of starting a new life in England; being loved by her perfect, blemish free, prince; or simply being free. She'd left her home, her friends and family for a man who was in love with another woman. A bitterness was beginning to creep inside and Ravi's words pricked like needles over her body. She wanted to hit him with a stick. A good fat stick with sharp splinters sticking out. She wanted to scream at him, kick and spit, but she did nothing. Her brain froze over with the shock that was Dimna. And laying like a zombie she asked in a mild little voice

'Do you still have contact with her?'

'No.' Ravi said drifting into the bathroom.

Mina looked down at the open album on the floor. Dimna looked up at her, smiling, laughing, and mocking. She scrutinised Dimna's plain face, her thin lips, her small eyes, her pointy nose, and her mousy brown hair. And she stared at her chunky white legs, skin whiter than bird shit.

'She's got awful knees,' shouted Mina.

Ravi walked up, with toothpaste foaming mouth, to examine the offending knees.

'What's wrong with them?'

'They're fat.'

Ravi laughed and reassured her with a pat on the head before returning to the bathroom to spit.

Mina turned the next page and saw another photograph of Ravi with his arms around Dimna's fleshy shoulders. In the next was a photograph of a different woman, prettier than Dimna, dressed in stylish clothes, sitting outside a Cafe, flashing a string of whiter than white teeth.

'Who's the woman in the pink coat?' Mina asked growing increasingly irritated.

Ravi returned in silk pyjamas striped emerald green and ruby red.

'Just someone I met in Paris,' Ravi yawned.

'Did you have lots of girlfriends before you met me?' Mina looked anxious.

'A few.' Ravi sat on the edge of the bed and set the alarm clock.

'Do you still think about them?'

Ravi started to laugh derisively.

'It's not funny,' objected Mina.

'You're so silly. Let's go to sleep. I'm tired,' said Ravi yawning again.

He climbed into bed, plumped up his pillow, rolled over and within a few minutes his breathing grew heavy and his lids opened slightly to reveal the whites of his eyes. Mina looked down at Ravi's face. His calm eyes, plump mouth and small nose, all cast in even shadow. There was no drooling mouth. No ruffled hair. He looked perfect. And suddenly she couldn't stand to look at him. Couldn't stand the tiny room, cheap net curtains and rotten old bed. Picking up the photo album she whacked Ravi on the shoulder shouting

'I shit on your love. I shit on you, I shit on you, I shit on you.'

She didn't really know what she was doing. It was instinctive to scream and pound her husband with that heavy album. With each blow, her pain seemed to ease a little so she hit him harder.

'Are you mad, woman?' said Ravi bolting up.

'Do you still love Dimna?' shouted Mina.

'No.' Replied Ravi turning away.

'Then why do you keep all these photos.'

'I don't know,' said Ravi lying down again.

'Can I throw them in the bin then,' hissed Mina.

'No, of course not. Just calm down and go back to sleep.'

Mina put down the photo album and pulled the covers over her. She couldn't sleep. Her body began to shake. Her eyes oozed with tears. Within minutes she felt Ravi's hands grope for a hint of breast. Disgusted, she flicked his hand away and listened to it flop indifferently to the side. As his hand moved across her thigh, up towards her breast she felt a volcano of anger swell inside. He'd screwed up her life and he was trying to touch her up. He could go to hell and she flicked his hand away once more. Ravi gave up and turned his back to her. The spot of skin where he'd touched her felt cold now. Staring into the dark, Dimna's face appeared in her head, going round and round giving her no relief. And in the night she got up and scrutinised the picture of Dimna with her white knees, thin lips and big hair. And she wondered, how could he love that when he has me? I was waiting for my wedding day. I never had a boyfriend. I was waiting for the right one. I could have married anyone I wanted. Who is he anyway? A half educated nobody. I have a degree, a Masters, a future.' But it was Mina who felt inadequate and desperate. It was she who was in need of Ravi and it was that need that scared her.

Ana listened to her mother tell the story of Dimna. It was a name she'd heard throughout her childhood. Dimna was Ravi's first true love. She was the one he was supposed to marry. She was the one who left Mina shattered and broken. Ana had seen a picture of her in the green photo album. Mina was right she had fat fleshy knees. She wasn't that beautiful. She looked plain and white. How could Ravi be in love with her? Was he in love with the idea of marrying an English woman? Where was she now? What was she doing?. Why couldn't Mina forget? She had a new life now. Perhaps it was because Mina loved to live in the past, rather than the now. The now didn't interest her, it was those who were no longer here, those who had died who were still in the present for Mina. It was those memories of the rivers, the roaming chickens, the dozy cows chewing grass, the women in the fields sifting through hay in the blaze of the sun that's what mattered to Mina. Ana watched as Mina curled into a ball and said to her mother 'you look distant' and Mina replied with a wistful look in her eye 'that's because I'm going back.'

Mina woke up the next morning to find Ravi gone. She stretched out in the bed. Tried to nestle down under the covers and rubbed her eyes, sore from no sleep. She felt like retreating into a comfortable dream but she couldn't relax. The sound of slamming doors, people's voices, creaks, footsteps, bangs, twittering birdies and stale thoughts interfered, forcing her to get up. She crept downstairs to the bank to see Ravi sitting behind a desk with his colleague. Dressed in his suit, white shirt and tie, he looked the part: a consummate professional. She tried to get his attention with a wave but he didn't notice her. She went back upstairs to see the photo album lying on the floor. Unable to help herself she began to pore over the pictures of Dimna before slamming it shut and throwing it across the room. It crashed into the leg of the bed. Growing slightly scared, Mina retrieved the album. There was a dent in the first page and the front cover was slightly scraped. She quickly put it back and tried to ignore the offensive item.

Sitting on the edge of the bed, not knowing what to do with herself Mina, for no particular reason, burst into tears; loud hearty sobs that left her exhausted. Feeling rather pathetic, Mina tried to get a grip. She washed her face put on some lipstick and feeling marginally better she began to rearrange things, make the room look nice but it still looked brown and dull. At midday she went back to bed. What was she supposed to do? Lie and wait for her husband. There were still seven hours to go. Ravi seemed to have settled straight into his nine to five job but what about her? If she stayed cooped up in the room with her wretched thoughts and Dimna's podgy cheeks she would go mad. Mina got up from bed with a sudden urgency and searched her suitcase for a book but she knew she'd left them all behind in a box under her bed in her hostel. She needed words. Words to squash out nasty thoughts. She needed to be home, to sit by her pond, to watch the ebb and flow of the water, the leafy carpets, and the light.

Mina lay on the bed and tried to sleep. Each time she closed her eyes she saw the green water of the pond and the trees standing on the edge waving their thick heads. It was bright, golden and too real. She could smell the leaf, the earth, and the dust in the air but when she opened her eyes she saw the four walls of the room, the dark, the brown. Screwing up her eyes once more she tried to make the images come. They didn't come. Just faint echoes of what she saw before.

Glancing at the clock it was 4.30. Still light. Still time. She draped herself in a pretty cobalt blue sari and ran out in search of a tree, a pond, some green. She hadn't walked far, only down the road. There was not much to see. A stray banana skin lodged in a crack, a half empty bottle of milk, a scattering of cigarette ends, a crisp packet washed up with leaves, a half eaten chicken leg, a crushed can of lager. She walked by the grocers at the bottom of Holfield road. Saw a little man struggling with a bag bursting with onions. The shop front read 'Butt's Gro ers.' The C was missing, the white paint no longer white. She saw the hacked holes in the road, patched over with slappings of tar.

Then she came to a dark and narrow alleyway that sucked her in. There was graffiti sprayed big and bold on the wall with a hole the size of a small fist. A hole that no one seemed bothered to patch up. She continued to walk until a black face splattered in white appeared from the shadows. Mina gasped but realised that it was only paint. She watched the man waddle round the corner dressed in dungarees that settled half way down his butt. She continued to walk. Walked past a skip overflowing with stink and rot. This was her new world and it wasn't pretty it was drab. Where was the light, the warmth, and the colour? Feeling the cold of fear that comes from unfamiliarity she quickly turned back. She wanted to run but in her sari she could only shuffle in short fast steps. And when she saw the clean facade of the bank she ran all the way up the stairs to find Ravi sitting on the bed reading the paper.

‘Where have you been?’ he asked irritably.

‘I wanted to buy a mango but I couldn’t find any,’ was her spontaneous lie.

‘At this time?’ Ravi spun around, his face amazed.

‘Yes,’ she replied standing by the window looking out at light in the sky. There was not a single tree, a hint of water or green and she sighed.

After a long silence Ravi said 'There's a grocers down the road, why didn't you go out and buy some food instead of a mango.'

'I don't know what to buy.' Mina raised her voice slightly

Ravi looked genuinely shocked. 'What do you mean?'

'I said I don't know what to buy.'

Looking up at the ceiling in despair Ravi responded ‘well you were going to buy a mango, what about vegetables, rice, chicken.'

He paused 'you don't you know how to cook? I learnt to cook when I was eleven. I had to feed my brothers and sisters. No one taught me, I just learnt by myself. Now I can cook twenty, thirty, forty dishes no problem.'

'My mother never brought me up to be a housewife,' she replied 'She brought me up to have a good education and a career. I've never been near the kitchen in my life.'

Ravi looked dismayed 'So who's going to cook then?'

'Why don't you get one of your English lady friends to cook?' snorted Mina.

Ravi flared his nostrils at his wife. 'Listen, there are no servants to cook and clean your arse here!'

Mina glared at Ravi but he just stomped past her out the room. She heard his footsteps on the stairs and the slamming of the front door. Standing by the window, she watched Ravi walk briskly into the grocer's store. The storeowner, an Asian man with a dome of a tummy, greeted him like an old friend. And she watched as Ravi sniff red chillies one by one, molested onions and squeezed the odd-looking veg. He returned fifteen minutes later with two bags of bulky shopping.

'Come with me,' Ravi grunted and Mina followed him reluctantly into the kitchen.

'OK I'm going to show you how to make rice.'

'I know how to make rice,' grunted Mina.

'Go on then.'

Mina grabbed the rice bag and tried to tear it open with her teeth. After two minutes of wrestling with the stubborn plastic, Ravi intervened with a pair of scissors. She didn't say thank you, instead she began to pour the rice into a pan.

'Aren't you going to measure the rice first?' Ravi remarked.

'This is how I do it,' she snapped. Filling the pan with a gush of water she swirled her fingers around the rice before pouring out the excess. Losing patience Ravi shouted. 'What a waste. You're pouring half the rice down the sink. That's Basmati rice you know. It's not cheap. Come on let me do it.'

'No, I can do it,' said Mina turning the tap too hard. A sudden spurt of water sprayed onto her sari front leaving a small puddle on the floor.

'What the hell are you doing?' asked Ravi looking down. 'Look my socks are all wet.'

'I'm filling the pan,' Mina protested.

GUNGI BLUES

'But that's too much water,' said Ravi looking down at the mess at his feet.

'No it isn't. This is how my mother does it.'

'I thought you said you never went near the kitchen.'

'I did pleasure cooking during the holidays,' replied Mina firmly.

Walking up to the stove she turned on the gas. Ravi produced a box of matches from his pocket and struck a match.

'Here, you do it,' he said holding the burning match in front of her face.

She placed it near the stove and a flame soared up making her gasp. Ravi started laughing.

'So what are going to make with the rice?'

'Anything you like.'

'Well I fancy chicken, aloo and dhal. Can you make that?'

Mina went quiet as Ravi rolled up his sleeves and started to wash, de-skin and chop the chicken into small pieces. He measured out the dhal and placed the potatoes on the boil. Heating up some oil he stirred his onions with brisk confidence. Then he opened his spice packets one by one, pouring them carefully into individual white bowls. Mountains of yellow, umber, sienna and rust sat waiting. Ravi added a sprinkling of each colour to the pan and Mina examined the packets, trying to memorise the names: cumin, turmeric and mixed spice. Soon a pungent aroma flooded the kitchen.

In went the chicken. He tossed and stirred. Twenty minutes later he smashed up the potato added finely chopped onion and chilli. Then a teaspoon of this and that in his simmering dishes. Each dish he tasted, smelt and added salt here and there. Within an hour a meal was ready. The chicken was tender, the dhal fresh with coriander, and the rice fluffy. And all Mina could do was sit down and eat up.

Everyday Ravi went downstairs to work in the bank and Mina tried to play the role of housewife. She slipped out the world of books, grand concepts and formulae and entered a New World of frying fish and washing up. Her first real attempt to cook was making dhal. She spent half an hour cutting her onions, garlic, tomatoes and coriander. She spent another twenty minutes measuring the lentils and the water. All she had to do was let it boil. But when she tentatively lifted the lid to inspect her creation her dhal resembled a mushy brown pulp.

During the next fortnight Mina prayed to Allah for a culinary miracle and dived into the array of spices, lentils and chickpeas waiting in the kitchen cupboard. After a week of destroying pans, burning fish, overcooking and undercooking Mina felt increasingly inadequate in the kitchen but she refused to give up because then Ravi would have won. He'd think she was useless and she wanted to prove him wrong. She started to experiment, buying strange ingredients, weird looking vegetables, unusual fish, pheasant and duck. She stopped trying to emulate Ravi and created her own dishes. Her food simply evolved. She might have intended to make two dishes and ended up making five. Suspicious of cookbooks and finding scales too oppressive Mina simply added a pinch of this, a bit of that and used her nose as a guide.

When he returned from work, Ravi often found Mina deep in a mess of boiling pans, unwashed plates, marinating fish, soaking meat, half cut veg, sniffing over her dishes, muttering to herself, contemplating the missing ingredient. But at the dinner table Ravi still griped 'the floor's disgusting, my feet keep on sticking to it.'

Mina responded with 'does the food taste good?'

'Yes it's good.'

'Then shut up and eat.'

One evening she attempted a dish of curried duck with mashed aubergines and fried rice. Using every pan at her disposal the tiny kitchen became cluttered with half cut vegetables, pans on the boil and duck skin on the floor. She sniffed at her dishes, before adding the missing ingredient, but if she was honest she was just blagging her way through. Trying to carry a pan in one hand and open the oven door with another, she burnt her thumb on the metal rack. Then struggling to set the table with her left hand, a plate slipped from her oily fingers smashing onto the floor. It wasn't any old plate; it was the one with pretty purple flowers and gold edging.

When Ravi found Mina sweeping up the broken remains he asked sadly 'How did you do that?'

'I just dropped it,' Mina replied as she chewed on a slither of duck.

'Why can't you be more careful?' Ravi stared at the fragments lying in the dustpan, mixed up with flecks of duck, vegetables and dirty dregs.

Mina turned away and sulkily dished out a dollop of rice and curried duck drenched in fat. She watched Ravi inspect her culinary experiment. He sprinkled salt over the duck without trying it first but Mina stayed quiet, because she was too tired to make a fuss.

Is this the life of a married woman? She asked herself. Although Mina didn’t have any preconceptions, she never expected a life of dusting, washing, mopping, sweeping and shopping. In some ways life was simpler in Dhaka.

GUNGI BLUES

She used to get up, eat, study and sleep. She didn't have to think. Coming to Bradford with Ravi was supposed to fulfil her dream of a big romance in a foreign land. Dimna ruined all that and now she felt trapped in a web of negative thoughts that seemed to grow daily and make happiness seem like a remote concept.

Some days, the days she didn't fancy cleaning, she found herself outside, on the streets, roaming Bradford. Behind Holfield road was Busby's Department store; a grand old red brick building with revolving doors. The assistants at the make-up counter were all smiles with faces heavily caked in white powder. After Busby's Mina usually didn't know where she was going but she felt compelled to walk, to enter backstreets and those side roads. On Tuesday morning she ended up on Lumb Lane. She saw grey council flats, hanging saris blowing in the wind, a chicken leg lying on the street, crisp packets washed up with leaves and bloated jack fruit spilling onto the pavement. An English girl with white blond hair wearing jeans that were too tight and a top that clung to her bee sting breasts strutted past her. Another girl, a woman, a granny, Mina couldn't tell because she was hidden inside a cave of black, watching the world through a slit of light. She crossed the road and saw three boys with gelled up hair loitering by a car that was half white and half brown with rust. It had no tyres, no doors, no windows; it was just a shell. 'Hello nice pussy', they heckled, 'give us your number darlin'. Mina kept her head down, didn't dare look up in case she grinned and sped past the Cash and Carry filled with one thousand packets of toilet roll and sacks of Basmati rice. There was a sudden stink of onions and rubbish in the air. A kebab shop on the corner was buzzing with locals chewing on samosas laced with mint yoghurt sauce. The shop had a simple interior; blue tables, red lino floor and mirrored walls to give the place a more spacious feel. The owner stood behind the counter, his hair cropped short, his pallor shiny, his clothes worn and his teeth stained red from chewing too much Paan. The cheapest thing on the menu was 10p. Mina couldn't resist the 20p kebab rolls. Kebabs drizzled in yoghurt, sprinkled with green chilli, tucked in naan bread. The owner stared at his black Mercedes parked out front and Mina wondered how many kebabs he had to sell to buy it. Mina climbed up a steep road. When she reached the top she saw the city, the council blocks, patches of green, distant buildings and a scrap heap of junk. She saw a little old lady emerge from a disused hut. She was wearing a red jacket and slippers. She walked a few steps forward and then returned to her hut. Back and forth several times walking in tiny pin steps. Mina watched until a lump filled her throat and she couldn't watch anymore. She took one final look at the looming blocks, the sloping rooftops, the wonky windows and the crumble before turning back.

Mina took a detour down a side street and came across a line of sparkly sari shops; she stopped to gaze at the five mannequins in the window. Draped in shimmering greens, reds and blue silks, Mina admired the gold embroidered finish and the tiny red flowers dancing on the border. She looked up at the mannequin's round, pink cheeks, green eyes and long lashes. Then she peeped into the next shop, brimming with hundreds of tapes. The windows were plastered with posters of Bollywood stars; men with moustaches wearing tight white pants. A flurry of flute, a tink tink, followed by a high-pitched voice and a tabla beat blasted out of the shop. Mina paused to listen, shaking discreetly to the beat.

The shop next door sold nick-nacks. Anything from white plastic buckets to cheap leather sandals and gold nose rings. There was a butcher's opposite called 'Halal Meat.' A man, wearing a blood stained overall, emerged from a van with a carcass draped over his shoulder. Flecks of white fat dotted the purple flesh and Mina saw skinless hunks hanging from metal hooks in the van. The smell of raw meat mingled in the air and made her heave. She crossed over to the other side and saw an old man with a long grey beard wearing socks and brown sandals, an embroidered skull cap on his head and a crisp white punjabi. He walked steadily with his gaze fixed on his toes. He didn't notice Mina. He was too busy trying to make it to the mosque. At midday the sound of prayer drifted over Lumb Lane. Melodic, profound, guttural and solemn. Mina paused and thought of Nana praying in the front room.

There was something familiar about Lumb Lane. The smells, the sight of Jack Fruit lining the pavement, the men with their long scrags of beards, the women draped in black, the dogs pissing randomly at lamp posts, the peeling posters of film stars and the rotting rubbish laying abandoned in the middle of the street. The pinch, the peel and stink all smacked of back home.

Mina's walks made her realise that there was more to life than cooking and washing up. Without telling Ravi she enrolled at the local library. Slipped away there in the afternoon. Read anything from elementary Chemistry books to cheap romantic fiction to Thomas Hardy's Far From the Madding Crowd. Mina even called up for a Bradford University prospectus to check out the post-graduate courses. She could imagine attending that red brick university. She could imagine feeling at home amongst the thousands of books. Her brain was turning to jelly; she needed stimulation, she needed knowledge. She applied through UCCA to Leeds, Sheffield, Manchester and Bradford University; and she received a placed at Leeds to study Geology. Mina never took up her university offer, she just applied because she wanted to see if she was good enough to get in.

She never told Ravi that she was bored; she didn't have to. When he came home from work, Mina was usually curled up in bed with her head hidden under covers. At breakfast she was quiet, picking at her cereal. At dinner she was laconic, gazing out the window, dreamy eyed.

It was Friday, Mina's favourite day of the week. The day that Ravi handed over his pay cheque and she stashed it in her pillowcase. The sound of crinkling cash in her sleep made her feel secure and hopeful for the future. Friday was also the start of the weekend, the day Ravi reserved for them to take long bus rides up and down Bradford, to go for lazy boat rides on the lake. Saturday night was Mina's excuse to dress up in her best sari. It was the night she and Ravi treated themselves to a movie. Walking down Holfield Road into the town centre, Mina marvelled at the tiny lights dotted over the city and for a moment Bradford looked like a dazzling flash place. Descending the street, Mina saw the Odeon lit up in bright lights like a space ship standing tall next to the mighty Alhambra, shrouded in neon blue fuzz. Couples, tarted up in tight skirts, beehives, gelled black hair and polished shoes ruled the streets.

"A Wonder of Love" was showing that night and Mina examined the poster of the dashing couple, entangled in a deep embrace. The way they looked at one another showed true intimacy. This was going to be the real love story, Mina thought. Sitting next to one another, Mina and Ravi munched on their popcorn. Shot in stark black and white Mina was sucked into the tragic world of three beaten lovers. There was one scene when John was saying goodbye to Sophie. Mina had never seen an on screen kiss before and found she was unable to turn away. She observed how John and Sophie held each other, their flaying tongues and panting chests. John reassured her that he was coming back. Sophie watched from her window. Watched him walk away and there was fear in her eyes. Then Sophie met Greg and forgot all about John. Greg was Sophie's first love. He left her but then he walked back into her life and suddenly John seemed rather insipid and far too earnest for Sophie. Greg was the crazy sort, the sort that liked to shag in the forest at night. The love affair didn't last and Greg disappeared without telling Sophie. She tried to kill herself and it was John who discovered her semi conscious in a cold bath. It was quite clear that John loved Sophie more and that Sophie was still obsessed with Greg who had moved onto a stream of chicklets. By the end of the film Mina identified with John's consistent love. Sophie was fickle and Greg was weak and vain but definitely mysterious and sexy. There was something of Ravi in him and seeing all those writhing limbs Mina just wanted to lie in bed with Ravi in her arms. It had been too long since they'd touched one another. They'd been married now for two months and they still hadn't had sex. Ravi had tried a couple of times but Mina instinctively pushed him away and slammed her legs shut because it never felt right. That evening Ravi and Mina held hands all night. He even slipped in a surreptitious kiss that created a warm feeling at the bottom of her belly. As they walked, their bodies slightly colliding, fingers touching, Mina couldn't wait to get home.

When they got back to the room there was no raunchy striptease, no big build up. Mina just brushed her teeth, slipped on her night dress, climbed into bed, closed her eyes and waited because she didn't know what else to do. She knew Ravi was awake. She could hear the gentle rhythm of his breath. Ravi was sitting on a chair gazing at his wife. Examining her cheekbones, her plump lips, her eyes slightly sunken from too many light nights and her perfectly plucked brow. Mina knew he was staring at her but she pretended to sleep. Ravi stripped off and climbed into bed. She didn't stir. Holding her tight from behind Ravi began to rub his body against hers. It felt warm and close. His hands pulled at her night dress until it was way up by her neck. Climbing on top now he tried to slip it in. She felt the hard tip squeeze against her and Mina opened her eyes in shock. Ravi didn't stop. He pushed and shoved his way past her dry lips. All the way in now. And there was much exertion and silly writhing and Mina let out a succession of gasps but she was not quite sure what she was supposed to do or what she should feel. She wanted to be like Sophie gasping and panting but she lay like a lump letting out little whimpers of pain. There was no pleasure, only a strange sensation of being violated. Riding her hard now, Ravi stroked Mina's hair and kissed her face. His fingers were tender, his movements rigorous.

'Does it hurt?' he asked softly.

Mina shook her head but it did hurt. His slippery cock lump suddenly popped out and Ravi started to fumble with her hole.

Mina directed his fingers towards her and he slipped it back in. He was less gentle now because he was trying to keep it up. His breath grew heavy and he closed his eyes. His skin was hot with sweat. Mina watched, feeling nothing much inside. She saw a flicker of ecstasy across his face. Ravi opened his eyes, pulled it out and before they could even exchange two words he ran out to the bathroom. Mina heard the trickle of running water and waited. Ravi returned uninhibited in his nudity. He prowled around the bed, showing off his taut torso, his shapely bottom and Mina admired the thing that dangled between his balls. Brown pink and soft. Ravi jumped back into bed and patted Mina on the belly moving his hands down to her hole. Mina felt his fingers delve deep. He looked down at his fingers, slightly moist from her juice, and Mina watched him examine them closely. Leaping up he stripped back the covers and looked down at Mina's wide-open legs. Her night dress was still high up around her neck exposing her breasts, wet with sweat.

'Why isn't there any blood?' Ravi stared down; apart from a few stray pubic hairs the sheet was white.

'I don't know,' Mina looked bewildered.

'There should be blood on the sheet if you're a virgin,' repeated Ravi growing slightly hysterical.

'Maybe it's because I use a temple to hide the blood' whispered Mina pulling the bed sheet over her bare breasts.

'What?'

'A temple breaks you in.'

Ravi grew quiet and said 'it doesn't matter just go to sleep.'

'It does matter,' said Mina trying to hide the hurt in her voice.

'No it doesn't. There's no blood. I over reacted. Go back to sleep.' Ravi switched off the light, climbed into bed and turned away from Mina. She was shocked by his reaction and all she could think was 'how could he even think I'm not a virgin? Dimna was no virgin. He's no virgin the bloody conservative bastard. I never touched a man, kissed a man, sniffed a man before I met him.' Mina felt rejected, unloved, like that Sophie character. What if Ravi divorced her? 'What if he didn't love her anymore?' Mina began to despair. Her despair turned to anger once more. Mina wrestled with rejection, fear and anger. The emotion swelled up in her throat, burning into hot tears. Ravi was awake, his eyes drifting from ceiling to carpet to curtains. The sobbing grew louder but he just let Mina cry herself to sleep.

The morning after Mina skulked around the flat with a face screwed up in frowns and scowls. She made soggy rice and sloppy dhal in protest and when they ate she avoided Ravi's eyes and only spoke to say 'Could you pass me the salt?' There was two weeks of grumpiness and sniping until Ravi began to try. He cooked her a meal of Coral fish, Mina's favourite and sang songs from Pakeezah, a classic Bollywood film, in her ear. But Mina just told him to 'shut up.'

Two weeks past with the same routine and Mina's face crinkled up as she looked at herself in the mirror. 'Cooking, cleaning, eating, shitting. This is my stupid life. What the hell am I doing? I'm mad. I had a scholarship to do my MSc and I walked out for what? I don't want to live in this bloody room. I don't want to be a bloody housewife. I don't want to rely on some bloody man.'

Mina beat her head against her hand for another two minutes, and then she picked at her teeth with a tooth pick. Trying hard to concentrate on the gum, random images filled her head. She saw herself on the bed, saturated in blood, with Ravi sitting beside her, looking smug. She saw herself in the kitchen tending to four pans. She saw herself wandering through the back streets of Bradford. Then Dimna appeared in her mind to irritate and Nana's sobbing haunted her. The images and sounds simply didn't stop because she thought her life was finished, that she was totally worthless.

That night as Mina turned over to sleep she felt a cold misery spread through her body and although Ravi tried to placate her with kisses and cuddles she remained unreceptive. In the night the images re-visited her. She saw Ravi sitting on that park bench kissing Dimna, caressing her white knees, whispering 'I love you' in her ear. She saw Dimna wearing a mini skirt and clingy top, squatting in the kitchen singing happily as she de-scaled fish. She saw them sitting at the dinner table laughing, eating and drinking red wine. And she believed it all until she woke up the next morning to see Ravi busily pottering around the room. Mina watched him from beneath the covers. Suddenly, he flipped back the sheet to expose Mina's hairy legs and half her bum. She angrily pulled down her pink night dress and Mina's grimace gave into a smile and a giggle.

After a meagre breakfast of a banana and a cup of PG tips they left their little room. Mina followed Ravi past the bus stop over the main road to a side street that led them to a pair of wrought iron gates. Beyond the gates was green grass and fat trees. She watched two kids rolling down the hill, screaming 'watch the dog shit'. She observed a mother hold back her son as he tried to run free. She saw an old woman walking her poodle and bulldog. She glimpsed a young couple, with their arms and tongues entwined, hiding in the long grass. Side by side, Mina and Ravi walked and then she saw it. A stretch of water. A pond of sorts with an island of hand planted trees in the centre. Ducks were swimming on the surface, fighting over crusts of bread, and Mina felt like stripping off and diving in.

Mina stepped into the boat, it wobbled nervously with her weight and as she plonked herself down water came up over the sides and splashed her feet. Ravi daintily hopped in and grabbing the oars they drifted along the pond edge. Mina didn't mind the leak in the boat or the damp. She just put her hand in the water and watched it ripple through her fingers. And for one hour she grinned and laughed. She forgot about Dimna, she forgot about cooking and she forgot about that poky room, until the boat trip came to an end and it was time to go back.

Mina went to bed with a little smile on her face after her dose of nature. Water and trees left her calm because they made her dream of her Pathuakali jungle, the paddy fields and lakes. She whimpered with the simple joy that memories bring and Ravi responded with gentle fingers. He stroked his wife's hair and kneaded her fleshy breasts. Half-asleep Mina was dreaming of drifting in that little boat. Ravi was singing to her and it was all too real with white butterflies in the air. When she opened her eyes she saw Ravi's naked body on top of hers and despite herself she responded to his full-blown kisses. Mina was a little less inhibited. She touched

Ravi's thighs and stroked his back. She tried to move, she tried to engage and she felt a little pang of something down there, very warm, like a rush of hot air through her whole body.

After that they made love at least once a week, usually at the weekend, when Ravi wasn't so tired. Sex started off with a kiss and a fondle. Ravi always took control riding his wife with a certain confidence. With time Mina grew bored being on the receiving end and pushed her way on top. She learnt how to move, give herself that hot rush and slowly began to enjoy the ride.

A fortnight later Mina woke up with stiff, heavy legs, stinging eyes and aching head. She wanted to close her eyes and fall into a soft comfortable dream but in the end she forced herself up. Queasiness in her stomach made her puke in the morning. She thought it was that old lump of fish she'd snacked on for lunch. It was only after days of throwing up in the sink that she went to the doctors for a urine test and that same evening broke the news to Ravi.

'You're pregnant' said Ravi rubbing at his face.

'I think so' replied Mina looking down at the bedspread.

'But how can you be pregnant?'

'Because we had sex.'

'Yes I know that but didn't you take precautions?' Mina began to pick at the loose threads on the bedspread.

'I told you to go on the pill remember' said Ravi running his hands through his hair. Mina only remembered Ravi leaving a box of tablets in the bathroom cabinet. He never consulted her he just expected her to take them.

'Don't you know you should have gone on the pill. Do I have to tell you everything? Don't you have any common sense? You're an adult aren't you?'

'I took them for two weeks.'

'Why the hell did you go off them?' he shouted raising his hands.

'Because the veins in my legs swelled up and I couldn't walk.'

'Oh.' Said Ravi rubbing his eyes. Calming down slightly. 'Are you sure you're pregnant?'

'I had a urine test this afternoon. It came out positive. The doctor said I'm pregnant.'

Wasn't being pregnant supposed to be one of the happiest days of your life? Wasn't it supposed to be a time to celebrate? It was their chance to make a little family. Instead she felt sombre as she looked down at the faded pattern on the bedspread.

' I didn't plan to have children for at least another five years. I want us to be settled, have a house, a car. I want to have a good position in the bank. In a few months, if I carry on working this hard I'll be a manager, then we can think about children.'

'So what are you saying?' Asked Mina staring at Ravi. He looked like a wreck, his hair was ruffled and there were bags under his eyes.

'I want us to postpone,' said Ravi catching Mina's eyes.

'But I'm already pregnant,' said Mina slamming her hands on the bed in frustration.

'You know what I'm saying,' said Ravi turning away.

'No I don't' said Mina banging her hands on the bed once more.

'Stop being silly.'

'I'm not being silly, I don't understand what you're saying,' said Mina chucking a pillow on the floor.

'Mina pick it up and stop being stupid. Listen I want you to go to a clinic and sort it out.'

'What?'

Lowering his voice Ravi said 'I want you to have an abortion.'

'You want me to kill my baby,' shouted Mina suddenly leaping up from the bed.

'Don't say it like that? God you're so over dramatic.' Ravi lowered his voice and walked up to the door as if he'd heard something.

'You want me to kill our child,' repeated Mina in a faltering voice.

'Keep your voice down. I think there's someone in the corridor. Let's talk about it tomorrow,' said Ravi in a loud whisper.

Mina grew hysterical and throwing herself to the floor she started to slap her face repeatedly until her cheeks blushed red. I cook, I clean, I do everything. What do you want from me, my blood?' Mina wailed.

'Why are you acting like a loony?' said Ravi massaging his head with both hands.

'Yeah I'm a loony. An oogy. A gungi,' shouted Mina recalling the times that Nana had dismissed her mother as mad to shut her up.

Ravi turned his back on Mina and opened his briefcase.

GUNGI BLUES

'What are you doing?' asked Mina watching Ravi in disbelief.

'I've got to sort my papers out.'

'What right now?' Mina began to claw at the bedspread.

'Look there's no point talking to you when you're screaming.'

'I'm not screaming,' screamed Mina and she stormed out.'

There was nowhere to storm to apart from the toilet. She sat in the dark, enduring the smell, clutching her head, rocking back and forth, crying, swearing, and beating her thighs. 'I hate men.' She said to herself. 'They don't respect us, they want to kill our children. I should run away from these awful men.' It was Ravi whom she hated at that very moment but she was too scared to admit it. She hated him for wanting to get rid of their first child. She should have told him how she felt but she didn't know how so she returned to bed where Ravi was snoring. She wanted to wake him up. Hit him. Shout at him. She'd been at that point many times before. It never did any good because she was the one who always felt like the loony.

The months trudged by, Mina watched her breasts expand, her stomach inflate with child and Ravi acted as if nothing was going on. They didn't talk about the baby, they didn't make plans, and the pregnancy just hovered in the background. It was only when Mina lay in the bath and saw her beast of a stomach bobbing merrily in the water that she fretted 'What if I'm a bad mother?' 'What if I can't do it?' 'What if the baby gets stuck?' Then she calmed down. Her mother bore seven kids into the world. It was in Mina's blood to have children

Apart from her growing bump and heaving bosom, life resumed as normal. Returning from the local grocers, weighed down with two bulky bags of shopping, Mina saw a young man, tall and slim with dull brown hair, staring at her. She thought nothing of it until he was standing right beside her.

'Can I help you with your shopping?' he asked gently.

'No I'm fine,' replied Mina looking straight ahead.

'You're very beautiful, yer know.'

Mina tried to ignore him.

'Can we go somewhere for a chat and cup of tea.' He bumbled awkwardly.

'I'm married,' Mina spluttered.

'I don't wanna marry yer I just wanna to talk to yer.'

GUNGI BLUES

'Can't you see?' Mina pointed to her bump but the man looked bemused. Rolling her eyes Mina shouted 'I'm pregnant.'

'It doesn't matter' said the man growing more desperate. 'I don't wanna have yer kids I just wanna go out with yer.'

'Sorry, bye,' Mina couldn't believe he had the audacity to ask her out.

'Listen luv, seeing you has made my day.'

Mina softened, started to smile shyly and the man grinned.

'See I made yer smile.'

Turning the corner into Holfield Mina was still smiling. When she opened the flat door she found Ravi sprawled out on bed reading the paper. Mina was bright eyed even though the shopping bags were cutting into her hands.

'You know what just happened,' said Mina excitedly.

'What?' replied Ravi casually.

'A man tried to pick me up.'

'Very nice, I'm very happy for you,' said Ravi turning a page of his paper. Ravi tried to act indifferent but inside he was rather aggravated by the undue attention his pregnant wife was receiving.

'Anyway if you go out dressed like that what do you expect?' Mina looked down. She was wearing a full-length sari and coat. The only naked flesh on show was her toes.

'What do you mean?' asked Mina.

Growing more irritated Ravi said 'Look, I think it would be better if you didn't go out so much?'

Mina was getting angry now. Walking was perhaps her only real past time. She thought Ravi was being irrational and acting jealous for no reason.

'It's not my fault if men look at me.'

Ravi started to unpack the Baked Beans and lentils.

'You did hanky panky with Dimna and that's OK but I'm not allowed to walk on the street.'

Ravi walked out without a word and Mina drifted into the bathroom. She stared at the face looking back at her. The face in the mirror was calm, with even features, nose slightly pink from the chill, hair messy with curls bouncing against her cheeks. 'I can't help it if I'm attractive,' she thought. 'It's not my fault if men look at me.' She peered into the mirror. Her pupils were circles of pure black and within that black were an infinite array of shapes. She could see herself in the iris, all distorted and compressed. She could see the bathroom. The curtains. There were dots of light in her eyes. Thick lines of lash. She noticed a pool of black under her left eye formed over years of late nights and insomnia. Mina shifted onto the second eye, bigger than the first, with a myriad of veins melting into abstract patterns on the ball then to the eyebrow straight and unkempt. There were nine creases in her brow. She counted them all. She moved to a slither of black. The black crept onto the arch of the nose; it curled and twisted. She moved down to the upper lip, crusty and tight with concentration. The bottom lip was broken into flecks of light and cracks of dark. Her lip fell open and three white doors that were her teeth peeped out into the dark. A tiny mole provided distraction. Then there was the hair. Too much hair everywhere. In that face Mina suddenly saw all the stuff that people hide away behind a layer of thin make-up, fragile smiles and feeble jokes. She didn't seem that attractive anymore. Mina looked down at her bump. Large and imposing. Round and dome like. She felt scared, happy, depressed and fat all at the same time. 'At least I'm healthy' she thought and stroked her tummy for solace before returning to the kitchen to pack her fridge with frozen chicken legs.

Rimi

Two weeks later Mina was rushed into hospital. She'd gone into town to return some library books. As she perused the shelves Mina collapsed and lost consciousness. When she re-opened her eyes she was in a white hospital room. The smell of disinfectant tickled her nose. A sudden piercing pain made her cry out for Ravi. After twelve hours of heaving, sweating and swearing, Rimi emerged, fist first, at 7:12 p.m., on 25 April 1970. Thrusting her arm up Superman style, in a hurry to discover life, Rimi ripped Mina's vagina. After seven stitches Mina lay alone in the hospital room waiting for the return of her baby. She looked around at the shiny floor and the bare white walls.

Her bed was positioned bang in the centre of the room, too far from the window to see the uninspiring view. The sterile bed with itchy sheets made Mina squirm in discomfort. Some twenty minutes later a trim nurse appeared with a tiny bundle held casually in one arm. The nurse promptly deposited the baby in Mina's arms and left. Holding the tiny thing, frightened of hurting her, Mina looked down at its soft swollen face. It was a rare maternal moment that Mina savoured before Ravi crashed though the double doors and startled Rimi into a loud bawl.

Mina smiled at her flustered husband.

'Boy or girl' Ravi asked anxiously.

GUNGI BLUES

'It's a girl' Mina beamed at the screaming brown face, right fist clenched, body twitching. There was a warm happiness that spread though her body when she looked down at her baby.

'A girl,' Ravi repeated failing to hide his disappointment.

Mina was still fatigued after the trauma of spreading her legs and having this living thing explode out her being. She chose to hide her feelings, swallow her anger and cradle Rimi close.

'Have you sent a telegram home?'

'No, what's the point,' said Ravi not bothering to take a look at his new daughter.

Mina understood. Ravi wouldn't send a telegram because the baby was a girl. That wasn't good news so why waste the money. Feelings of failure dissipated Mina's happiness but her grip didn't loosen. She held her little baby even tighter; tight enough to make Rimi cry.

With not enough room for a cot Rimi slept in between Mina and Ravi. It was cramped and uncomfortable and they endured their first week of sleepless nights and no sex. Ravi changed the occasional nappy when he was around, burped Rimi and patted her to sleep. He covered her bottom with the blanket after she kicked it off and lay awake to watch Rimi smack her lips. While Ravi worked from eight until late, Mina was left holding the baby.

At first she tried to carry on as before. She took Rimi to the library, tried to have a pleasant read until Rimi began to scream and they were politely kicked out. Mina tried to get on with the job of motherhood and settle into a new life of changing nappies, sterilising bottles and meeting the fastidious eating habits of Rimi. She painstakingly pureed banana, mashed up carrots and pounded fish into smartie size mouthfuls. Half the time Rimi spat her food out. Half the time Mina paced up and down trying to think up ingenious methods of getting her to sleep, most of which failed.

The bags under her eyes grew larger and she often didn't bother to brush her hair, some days she just stayed in her night dress only getting dressed if she really had to. When she finally did get Rimi to sleep Mina would lay down on her bed, close her eyes and dream. She didn't have sweet dreams. Negative thoughts haunted her. Why hadn't Ravi celebrated the birth of his little girl? Feelings of wanting to be boy returned because being a girl was worthless.

GUNGI BLUES

Mad Manchester

Three months after Rimi's birth Ravi was transferred to Manchester. It was time to move from that flat. Half empty milk bottles had become ornaments along the skirting boards. Nappies washed and used lay piled up, toys littered the floor; there was no room to move, no room to breathe. Manchester would provide new opportunities miles from the cramp and damp of Bradford. They moved into a flat above the bank on Wilmslow Road. It was smaller than 13 Holfield Road with bare floorboards, no curtains, one small window, a single bed without a mattress and one wardrobe.

Mina walked towards the window, drawn by the sound of traffic and people's voices. She saw orange double-decker buses chug by. Bright neon lights flashing above restaurants; reds, greens and blues of silk saris adorning mannequins that looked like movie stars; and stacks of vegetables, chillies, tomatoes, onions and wrinkled aubergines. This was Rusholme, home of the curry houses, grocery stores and sari shops that stretched a mile long.

It was Mina who discovered 6 Whitebrook Road. She overlooked the weeds in the garden, the flaking paint, the tininess of the rooms, the searing crack in the wall and the lopsided cupboards. The first thing she did was knock on the wall, the sound was low and deep. She ended up in the main bedroom looking down at the lawn that stretched long and wide. There was one lone oak tree with a thick gnarled trunk. The grass was overgrown and the rockery consisted of two rocks. Still, it was a solid little house and cheap. That evening Mina told Ravi 'I've found our house.' They made another visit the following Saturday as a whole family and Ravi fell for the Conifer in the front garden and saw the potential within those walls, Ravi and Mina bought 6 Whitebrook Road for three thousand quid.

A week after they moved in Ravi decided to visit his new neighbours. He knocked on Miss Redfern's door. There was no answer. Ravi looked through the letterbox and saw Miss Redfern's tall frame dart across the kitchen. He knocked again. Miss Redfern eventually undid the latch, poking her long nose around the door.

Ravi stretched out a hand but Miss Redfern didn't shake it. She was a tall lady with curly white hair. She wore thick-rimmed glasses and her teeth were yellow from smoking to many cigarettes. She wore brown leather slippers, a long pleated navy skirt and a cream blouse with a silver pendant around her neck. Ravi glimpsed her hallway. It was pristine with green carpets and freshly painted white walls. There was a little table by the stairway for her green telephone and there was no clutter.

Ravi looked up at her crosshatched face, tight thin lips, prescription glasses and smiled. A smile that was all teeth, dimples and sparkle.

She finally spoke 'Can I help you?'

'I just wanted to say hello.'

'Well nice to meet you, I really must go because my peas are boiling,' and she shut the door.

Ravi crossed the road to house number three. An old lady called Mrs Ballwinkle lived there. She didn't open the door even though Ravi saw her pale wrinkled face flicker behind her curtains. Moving on to house no five Ravi rang the doorbell where Mrs Harrison lived. A lady wearing soiled gloves and an apron opened the door. Her hair was scraped back in a bun on her head and Ravi noticed that she wore shoes without any tights. Ravi introduced himself and Mrs Harrison gave him a funny look. He tried to make small talk but Mrs Harrison said she was 'tied up with her tomatoes.' Mr and Mrs Walsh who lived right next door were the only ones who invited Ravi in for a cup of tea. Mrs Walsh was a rather elegant lady with blue rinsed snowy hair and a soft voice. Mr Walsh was a little rougher with his hard Belfast accent. Mr Walsh proudly showed Ravi their family tree, hand written in rich brown ink. Long and thin it stretched across their living room wall and Ravi marvelled at the fancy writing. After offering Ravi a second Bourbon biscuit, Mrs Walsh offered to babysit anytime.

When Ravi got home he found Rimi slumped on the sofa, sucking on a dummy that filled half her face. Ravi whisked Rimi up and hurled her puny body into the air. Growing delirious, Rimi's eyes rolled back. Mina complained 'I've just fed her, she'll be sick.' Ravi put her down and Rimi started to whinge.

‘If you are a naughty girl, I’ll go away and never come back again, now let’s go to Mummy.' Ravi whispered. Rimi's body squirmed in protest and she squealed as Ravi dropped her into Mina's silk lap. Small eyes, hamster cheeks and double chin were all Mina saw 'she doesn't really look like me' she said sadly.

'She's so small she doesn't look like anyone yet,' replied Ravi bursting a bubble of saliva on Rimi’s chin.

Ravi slipped Rimi into the pram carefully tucking in the blanket. He pulled a cotton cap over Rimi's black hair, stood back and admired his daughter.

Ravi watched his wife struggle to get the pram through the front door. Wearing a leaf print sari Mina strolled down the street pushing the black pram. Looking down at Rimi, Mina whispered 'I'm going to be the best mother,' but Rimi wasn't listening. She was staring up at the white clouds in the sky. Her eyelids began to droop and within five minutes the fresh air knocked her out.

Mina continued to walk. It was a quiet street, with a faint sound of yapping dogs, kids’ voices and the odd passing car. Mina examined the other semi-detached houses; the carefully planned rockeries, the trimmed hedgerows and neat front lawns. She looked into other people's windows and observed the porcelain statues, the potted magnolias and vases on ledges. She glimpsed wine-coloured sofas, coffee tables and a pair of swords hanging over a mantle-piece. On her way back she saw a pair of young kids chasing each other round a mustard Skoda, a young man lovingly washing his blue Mini and an elderly woman with swollen ankles walking her yapping Terrier but she didn't see another brown face.

Within a week of moving in Ravi settled into his job as deputy manager. The bank was located on Wilmslow road in between the Restaurant Sheezan and a grocery shop that sold everything from cotton buds and cornflakes to Lady Fingers, bunches of fresh coriander, birds eye red chillies, leafy spinach and boxes of mangoes, which were piled in crates outside the shop.

During his lunch break Ravi slipped into Sheezan for a couple of samosas. It had a lime green interior and fudge coloured carpets. Every square inch was filled with plastic table clothes and uncomfortable chairs in different shades of green. Paintings of Romantic English landscapes, waterfalls and mountains graced the walls. The owner's name was Ruben. Apart from the paintings he didn't spend a penny on the interior. He didn't have to. The place was always packed with locals, smoking their time away from noon until late, stuffing their face with chapatte and aloo. Ruben drove a second hand Jaguar. He wore a suit with a black tie. His shoes were polished and his cufflinks, pearl encrusted in gold, were cheap imitations.

'Bring the wife and the kid. Don't keep them locked up,' Ruben would laugh and Ravi laughed along with him.

Ravi was always too busy, working late, trying to make extra money through overtime. With that money he went into town to roam antiques shops hidden in grotty back streets. He came across one shop with three legged chairs and bits of wood spilling onto the pavement. Inside it was dark and mysterious and Ravi was enticed in.

A burst of colour on the wall caught his eye; an understated landscape with a brilliant misty sunset. It was by some obscure artist with a confident signature. Ravi stared at the painting trying to figure out how the artist blended the green, yellow and red into one perfect smudge. How did he make it so smooth? The light reminded him of home. The landscape was just a strip of purple. It might have been a field or a plot of land somewhere. He liked all things beautiful and this was a very magical thing; it was a painting of dreams and light. He checked the price tag. At five quid he couldn't really afford it but he bought it anyway. As Ravi walked out the shop, a flash of gold winked at him from a dark corner. It was the gold leafing of a teapot with ornate handles far too grand to make tea in. Ravi picked up the pot searching for cracks. It was flawless and the only blemish was the date 1521. Ravi picked up his purchases and was ready to walk out until, like a blond bombshell waiting at the bus stop, he saw it standing there; a green onyx table with delicate legs and tiny golden feet that almost walked. The onyx contained a sea of swirls and dancing ribbons of colour. Decorated on the edge of the table were small hand painted pieces of oval marble. Each oval contained a little story with faces, landscapes or figures wearing wigs riding white horses.

Ravi took a taxi home and got off at the corner so that Mina wouldn't know. When he unloaded his goods in the hallway Mina's face dropped. As Ravi caressed his teapot, he assured his wife that 'it didn't cost that much. That same evening he set to work arranging his bargain goods. The painting looked perfect in the front room, the onyx table matched the green curtains and the teapot took centre stage on the windowsill. Mina bought a few candles and arranged them in cheap coloured glass pots. During quiet evenings, when Rimi was snoozing in her cot and Ravi was still at work, she lit her candles, lay down on the floor and watched the coloured patterns flicker across the wall.

With Ravi's second pay cheque he bought a Y reg. VW Beetle. It was rusty white and if you looked really close there was a dent in the bonnet.

Mina slipped out of smelly cotton and draped herself in green silk with embroidered ducks. In a frilly frock dotted with yellow splodges Rimi bounced up and down on Mina's knee. And Ravi wore a black suit, a deep purple shirt and shades. It didn't matter that the sky was overcast and grey. Squeezing into the VW it croaked with the excess weight. Ravi stuck in his key. The engine spluttered. He stalled. He started her up again, gently this time, and they sped off down Whitebrook Road.

Ravi caressed the steering wheel and Mina enjoyed the breeze that was messing up her hair. Rimi was gurgling excitedly trying to grab the gear stick and Ravi suddenly broke out in song. Mina looked at him. He was handsome with movie star looks and a cheeky smile like John Lennon. Staring down at his right arm, Mina examined his skin, smooth and hairless like a Japanese man. Looking at that perfect piece of arm made her feel very lucky to have such a beautiful husband. Her feelings of luck quickly faded, replaced with indifference. It was strange, whenever she felt a pang of happiness something froze inside her and stopped her from enjoying the moment and she couldn't explain what it was.

They went for a drive once a month, usually at night, after work, around the residential streets of Fallowfield. It was supposed to be a family outing. If Ravi wasn't so tired they might go down Wilmslow road into Rusholme to soak up the bright neon lights and slow buzz. He would buy a box of sweet gelapi, bright orange and sickly sweet. By the time they reached 6 Whitebrook Road the box was usually empty, their fingers sticky and Rimi's baby pink bib covered in orange dribble.

Although they didn't have much money Mina used any spare pennies on plants. Within a month she'd bought a Cheese plant, a Money plant and a Yucca. They were weedy things at first. After weeks of daily watering tender green shoots sprouted up and whatever space in the house was invaded with shiny leaf and travelling stems. Mina often ended up in the back garden at night. There was a tree stump in the corner, crawling with fungus and smothered in moss. Mina squatted on that stump for hours just staring at the garden. In her mind though she created secret corners with climbing ivy, flowing fuchsias pink and red, wild bluebells, plump shrubs and shiny veg. At the bottom of the garden under the massive oak she had grown a little paddy field. It was only a patch of grass but to Mina it was her paddy field where one day a river might flow. The whole world was in her garden she thought. Her oak tree threw acid down on the puny grass but still the grass managed to grow in her little Pathuakali jungle.

Ravi returned from work, late on a Friday evening, to find Mina and Rimi were gone. In the kitchen there was steaming rice, simmering dhal and chicken bubbling in a pan but no trace of them. Then he looked out the window and saw Mina in her pink night dress and wellies digging in the back garden.

'What are you doing?' he yelled through the window.

'I'm planting., replied Mina happily.

'Where's Rimi?'

'She's right here.' Said Mina pointing at a patch of overgrown grass. Wrapped tightly in a white blanket Rimi lay half hidden in the long weeds. Ravi ran out and scooped up the sleeping baby.'

Ravi stood and watched his wife for a minute digging away without a single care. Her nose was running and she sniffed loudly in between digs.

He returned inside with Rimi. Sitting next to the bin was a bulging Asda bag with onion peel and banana skin hanging over the top. Then he saw a wooden bowl with peel, leaf and cores all thrown together in a mess of orange, green, reds and whites. He looked at the bowl with disgust.

Mina appeared and interjected 'that's going to be my compost. Any bones, veg, or fruit go in that bag. Nana made his own compost; he grew everything himself. Fresh tomatoes, sugar cane, potatoes and herbs.'

GUNGI BLUES

Ravi looked in the bag and his nostrils flared up in protest.

Mina spent her life in the garden and Ravi worked long hours at the bank. He soon learnt a Barisal community existed in Manchester. Ravi wanted to meet these people, befriend them and invite them to his new house for dinner. When Ravi broke the news to Mina that they weren't alone Mina groaned

'I don't want to entertain anyone, I don't want to cook, I want to be on my own in the garden.'

The first person he made contact with was Faisel, a friend of one of his colleagues at the bank. He lived in Burnage, not far from Fallowfield, with his wife and small son who had a penchant for breaking bricks. They went round for tea and Gelapi. As Ravi talked Mina's mind drifted to scenes of Dolu cutting coconuts in front of the ditch, her room flooded with light, the lane shaded by trees, the view of the rising sun from the roof and Nanu frying fish surrounded by giant pots. Faisel's wife kept on looking at Mina with her narrow eyes. She was a stodgy character with a sour mouth and fleshy fingers. They left after an hour and Ravi insisted that they all come to dinner. Mina rolled her eyes and as they walked to the bus stop she became grumpy.

'Why did you have to invite them? We haven't even unpacked yet.' Ravi ignored her. They stood in silence and watched as a small man came running towards them. He was smiling and waving. Mina observed that he was wearing trousers that were too short and a school like blazer. The lean young man was slightly out of breath. His face was slim, he had a dignified nose and his skin was rough like towel. He saw the repulsion in Mina's eyes. His skin was covered in spots like sponge cakes filled with too much cream. In an attempt to improve his skin when he was a teenager he soaked cotton wool in Dettol and gently dabbed his freshly burst spots. He listened to the sizzle and felt the ice cream of his skin being scooped away to leave gaping holes. But his skin saw no improvement and just mushroomed with a fresh layer of spots. Put off by Mina's eyes, the young man turned to Ravi and still gasping asked 'Are you Ravi?'

Ravi nodded.

'My name's Amit Bai, I'm a friend of Faisel's. He told me you were coming, I came as fast as I could. I didn't want to miss you. I'm from Barisal too you see. You know where the big red church is in Barisal, well our house is just opposite. Do you know it?'

Ravi was touched that the young man had run all this way to say hello and patted him on the back warmly. Mina was more reserved and stared at his ridiculous trousers

'Are you studying?' Ravi asked.

'Yes.' Amit Bai nodded proudly. 'I'm studying engineering at Salford University.'

Their faces were alive, their body language animated. Ravi recognised the loneliness in Amit Bai's eyes, a loneliness that comes from trying to survive in a foreign land. The bus arrived and there was no time to explain away the roughness of his cheeks or the short length of his trousers. Amit Bai smiled a warm brown smile, from too much Gelapi and not enough Colgate, and waved goodbye but Mina had gone straight to the back of the bus with her eyes focused sharply ahead.

'Get my number from Faisel and call me,' said Ravi waving from the bus.

Amit Bai watched the bus turn a corner. He went back to Faisel's house and asked for Ravi's number. He finished off the Gelapi and two cups of tea then he caught a bus to his hostel carrying two mangoes and his text books in a plastic bag. He walked slowly. He was in no rush. There was nothing to return to apart from an empty room. His room was tiny with a single bed in the corner, a desk and a lamp. Pulling a plate and knife from an open draw Amit Bai began to de-skin the mango. He slurped up the sticky slithers and soon sucked the bone dry. Opening up his thick textbook he settled down to study. His eyes refused to focus and shifted to the grey concrete blocks outside.

Amit Bai's father was one of the first batch of Commerce graduates from Dhaka University in 1926. It was natural that Amit Bai would follow his father's footsteps into education. They lived in a big white house on a busy stretch of lane where rickshaws and carts whizzed past. From his roof top you could see the lake where women washed clothes and pots, the road where people spat and children played and the Bengali Christians filing in for prayer every Sunday. Amit Bai studied hard but his grades didn't come easily. He thought it was because his parents were first cousins. He'd read somewhere in a eugenics book that inbreeding can lead to brain deficiency. Out of all his brothers Amit Bai did well enough to obtain a place to study in England. It was his dream to come to England, get a good degree and a well-paid job. He would have preferred the prestige of Oxford University but he never achieved the grades so he settled for Salford. Barisal was a small district. People quickly found out where people migrated to and Amit Bai found out about Faisel. He was his only point of contact in the new land. When he arrived in England he discovered baked beans and runny eggs. He quickly became homesick for his mother's cooking and the good life he had in Barisal playing cricket with his friends until last light. And in the night he saw his father sitting on a little stool on the porch reading the Koran or some book. He saw his long white beard, his body slightly tilted to the left and his green eyes. He was wearing a checked lungi and a white punjabi and Amit Bai missed his deep voice, his wise words and gentle pats. He missed his mother, the way she sat in the sunlight rocking back and forth. He missed her white silver hair, her skin thin, wrinkled and brown. Her eyes big and bright like some kind of exotic bird. And he missed his father's room where the light streamed in leaving golden patterns on the floor where he used to read and watch the people from the balcony.

Giving up on his books Amit Bai sat on his bed and watched the minutes tick by. At six o'clock it was time for food. Amit Bai queued up behind the long line of students and stared at the sloppy beans, thick chips and sweaty eggs heaped up on his plate. Amit Bai, sat at the end of the long dining table and forced himself to eat. No one talked to him. He wasn't interested in making conversation because he was too busy trying to keep his food down. Then he returned to his room, picked up his HB pencil and struggled with his technical drawing. His lines didn't connect and his perspective was wonky. Art wasn't taught at his school in Barisal, only maths, science, Bangla and English. He grew frustrated, broke his pencil in two and went to bed.

Unable to keep up with his lectures, Amit Bai found himself going to Faisel's house. It wasn't for the company it was just to speak Bangla. Speaking his mother tongue was some comfort. It was frustrating trying to speak English. He could never find the right words. On some evenings Ravi and Mina were there. Ravi was always animated and cracking jokes, which made Amit Bai laugh. They seemed to have so much in common, the same humour, the same positive view of life.

Amit Bai was retuning to his hostel one rainy afternoon. It was one of those grey, cold windy afternoons where all you want to do is shut the door and sleep. But he decided to visit 6 Whitebrook Road instead. He knocked timidly on the door. Mina answered carrying Rimi in one arm wearing a rather old sari. Her hair was loose and she wasn't wearing any makeup. Amit Bai could see she was embarrassed by the way she refused to look him in the eye as if she was trying to hide her naked face. Amit Bai was very gracious and asked

'Babi, is Ravi in?'

'No he's at work,' Mina was abrupt. She didn't invite him in and closed the door in his face. She didn't think Ravi needed any more friends and she was annoyed that Amit Bai hadn't rung beforehand.

Amit Bai decided to visit Ravi at Habib Bank. Even though he was working Ravi took time to sit with his new friend and talk for five minutes.

'Come to the house for dinner next Tuesday,' Ravi insisted.

Amit Bai was a little hesitant 'Are you sure Babi won't mind?'

Ravi looked surprised 'Mina loves entertaining. Please come. They slapped each other heartily on the back and Amit Bai was already excited about the invitation..

Amit Bai arrived in his best suit with an offering of Cadbury's Milk Tray. Shimmering in blue silk, with her hair tied up in a bun and her lips laced with red lipstick, Amit Bai was struck by Mina's transformation. Ravi welcomed Amit Bai like an old friend. The house swelled with the aromatic smells of Ravi's cooking. By evening they stuffed themselves with chicken smothered in rich hot sauces, fried aubergine, potato cakes drenched in oil and spicy fish that made the house reek. Rimi clawed at Amit Bai's trouser leg until he picked her up. She happily sat on his knee listening to them talk well into the night. That night marked the beginning of a friendship that Mina couldn't stop.

Ravi and Amit Bai could be seen walking down Whitebrook Road, looking dapper and dashing in their pencil thin trousers and short neat haircuts. From behind they looked like brothers. From the front they didn't look anything like one another. After a couple of months of hanging out, they both grew thick sideboards that concealed their cheeks and developed bellies from eating too much rice and sweet meats. They became two chubby blood brothers. Ravi placed several photographs of them on the telly. In one photo Ravi and Amit Bai were standing in the kitchen with their sleeves rolled up. In the other they were sitting on the sofa wearing shades and white flares, like Elvis except without the glitter.

Over the months the three of them led a life of chat, food and changing nappies. If Mina needed a lie down Amit Bai took care of Rimi, fed, bathed and patted her to sleep. Amit Bai was either in the kitchen washing up, hoovering the stairs or chopping the onions for Mina while she sat poring over a pile of thread, needles and cloth. She was trying to make some money on the side through sewing, even though she wasn't particularly good. Money was so tight that Mina put an ad in the local paper for a lodger. The phone didn't ring for a week. Mina was about to give up until one afternoon she received a call from a man with a deep gruff voice like a bear. As Mina explained that the room was very tiny the man interrupted her and asked

'What colour are you? Black?' You're a Paki aren't you?' and the man hung up.

The slam of the phone rang in her ear and Mina was in shock for about a minute. Then she promptly removed the ad and invited Amit Bai to stay instead. His halls were closed over the summer break and he was a very good baby sitter. Amit Bai had already accepted an offer from Faisel to lodge at their house but when Mina suggested he stay with them he jumped at the chance and moved out of halls within the week.

GUNGI BLUES

Mina was washing up and Ravi was drinking a cup of tea. His face gaunt, his skin grey green, he looked overworked and underfed. There was something Mina was waiting to spill but couldn't find the moment. She'd known now for a month. If she stayed quiet it might go away, she thought. Mina swished her hands in the tepid water playing with the suds. There was no easy way to say it. She knew Ravi wouldn't like it. She knew he'd wrinkle up his nose and frown. And then she took her hands out the water and came right out with it.

'Ravi I'm pregnant again,' Mina watched Ravi's face crease up.

'What?'

'I'm pregnant again,' she turned back to the sink to avoid his eyes.

'You're joking. What about the cap?'

'It didn't work,' she said slapping the water like a child.' Do you want me to get rid of this one too?'

'I never said that. Amit Bai is in the other room so keep your voice down,' whispered Ravi.

Speaking calmly and softly Ravi said 'we really can't afford another kid'.

Mina threw the pan back in the water and said bluntly, 'don't worry we'll find the money.'

'I'd love to have another baby, really' said Ravi unconvincingly. Mina cut him off before he could continue.

'There's never a right time to have kids. It just happens. We're not robots. We had sex, I got pregnant, there's no point saying 'we can't afford it.' If we waited for the 'right time' we'd never have any children.'

Ravi didn't respond because mid way through he escaped into the sitting room. Mina heard raucous laughter as she stomped upstairs to the bedroom. Rimi was fast asleep; her little face tranquil, her breathing full of snuffles and the occasional spurt. Mina felt calm just by looking at her. Proud that she had produced this little bundle. Mina sat by Rimi because she'd already been sick in the morning and she was terrified that Rimi might vomit again so she prayed that Rimi would be healthy and alright. Mina noticed that the wardrobe door was open. Split in two halves, the top shelf was for Ravi's clothes the bottom one for hers. His jumpers and shirts all neatly folded in three piles, so perfectly formed she felt like messing them up. Mina's clothes melted into a heap. A melange of knickers, grey bras, odd socks and laddered tights that needed to be chucked. Mina closed the wardrobe; she didn't want to be reminded of their fundamental incompatibility. She stared at her dressing table, covered in half empty bottles of lotions, old clumps of tissue, dust and hair before climbing into bed.

GUNGI BLUES

Mina was ready to go to sleep. She couldn't settle and lay with her eyes open, irritated by Ravi, irritated by the chaos in the wardrobe, the mess of her dressing table and the cardboard box that had been lying dormant under her dressing table for over a year. Mina pulled out the box and tore off the masking tape. She discovered a few books, a green leather bound photo album that looked familiar and an A4 brown folder stuffed with a bunch of old papers. Curious she tipped out the contents. Receipts, bank statements, an old train ticket and letters still preserved in their envelopes. Two of them were from Barisal. She recognised the thin blue paper with the zigzag patterned edge, the foreign stamps and the musty smell of spice and heat. The third was in a fresh crisp envelope, not worn and crumpled like the others. Written in Ravi's hand the letter was addressed to Dimna. Mina froze when she saw the name, a name that triggered fear, loathing and dread. After five long minutes of staring she opened the letter and slowly began to read.

25 September 1970

Dear Dimna,

I hope you are well and happy. I worry about you and think about you every day. I hate to think that you are sad and sitting alone somewhere under a tree. I've wanted to call you but I just didn't dare. It's easier to write. I know I should have written ages ago. Anyway, I'm writing now.

I live in Manchester and work at a bank. I drive a VW Beetle and live in a lovely house. It has three bedrooms, two living rooms and a massive garden with rose bushes and Conifers. I've filled the house with oil paintings and antiques. I found this beautiful onyx table for the front room. I just wish you could see it. Maybe you will one day?

I'll be honest, I've missed you and I still think about you. I hope you think about me now and then. Even though things didn't work out I'm glad we met. Are you married or seeing anyone? Let me know what's going on in your life and stay in touch.

Much love Ravi

Mina re read the letter and checked the date once more. These were recent words. There was no mention of Rimi, born 25 April 1970, no mention of his wife. They didn't exist in Ravi's pretty hand painted picture of Conifers and rose bushes. In his world he was a bachelor living it up with his flash car, his onyx table and fake Rodin's. Why did he ask if Dimna was married or not? Why had Ravi written to her when they were happily married with child? How could he do this to her? Mina suddenly felt worthless. Something was broken inside her. Mina wanted to run away from Manchester. She wanted to jump, sink and fall. She wanted to disappear fast from this life.

GUNGI BLUES

Too busy chatting with Amit Bai to notice the time, Ravi didn't come to bed until one in the morning. Mina had lain awake all this time waiting for him. She watched him feel his way over to Rimi. She began to wriggle in her cot, smacked her lips, flicked an imaginary fly from her ear, rolled over, flipped off her blanket and lay with her legs sticking defiantly in the air. Stroking her thick black hair Ravi re-arranged the blanket, tucked her in and then got into bed. Ravi was just getting comfy, settling down to sleep, before Mina asked in a cracking voice

'Ravi, are you still in touch with Dimna?'

'No,' Ravi said wearily.

'Well why are you still writing to her then?' Mina said coldly.

Ravi didn't answer.

'Why didn't you mention your wife and kid, hey?' Mina's voice was growing louder.

'Shhh, will you, Amit Bai will hear.'

'I don't care if he hears. How could you write to her? It's like we don't exist.'

'I didn't send it OK. Dimna wrote to me months ago, she was in a bad way and I just couldn't tell her about you. When I talked to her she seemed so low

I was afraid that if I told her I was married she might do something stupid, harm herself of something. I know she still has feelings for me and I couldn't take the risk.'

'So you saw her.'

'No she wrote to me.'

'You said you talked to her.'

'What does it matter, the letter meant nothing. I didn't even send it in the end. I'm sorry.' Ravi leant over and tried to kiss his wife but she turned away in disgust.

'I said I'm sorry, what more do you want?'

'Go to hell,' Mina screamed.

Ravi muttered and rolled over to sleep.

Hearing Ravi sleeping drove Mina crazy. She tutted and grunted all night but Ravi didn't budge. 'What a bastard,' she thought. 'How could he sleep? It's not right. I'm a mess and he looks happy. He's probably dreaming about Dimna.' Mina could feel her emotions churn. She didn't want to cry. She held those tears back and it was only at four o'clock in the morning that her eyes finally gave in. Mina woke up to discover that both Ravi and Amit Bai were gone. Rimi was jumping up and down in her cot demanding attention. Mina trudged over, lifted the baby out the cot and put her on the floor. Sitting on the edge of the bed she watched the box in the corner. She watched it for at least five minutes. Then she got up and searched for the letter. Mina wanted to read it one more time but it was gone. Maybe Ravi had other letters stashed away in secret corners, she thought. Maybe he had a whole pile of love letters crammed in a shoebox somewhere.

Obsessed with the box, the letter and Dimna, Mina didn't notice Rimi sitting in the corner. Rimi was unusually quiet and still. Something caught her attention under the bed. She started to crawl towards it. Mina's foot was obstructing so she pinched Mina's toe to make it go away. Mina yelled out in pain and that's when she saw the fluff sticking out of Rimi's nostrils. Rimi started to cry and tried to crawl away. Mina grabbed her legs and Rimi stared in Mina's eyes looking slightly terrified as she plucked out the fluff balls with tweezers, before setting her free. Rimi quickly crawled off towards an old shoe but something twinkled in the carpet. Mina was lying on the bed in a phlegmatic state while Rimi was going to eat that twinkling star. She put it into her mouth. Her lip split open. A glob of blood trickled down to stain her bib. Rimi laughed a contagious cute giggle that made Mina turn round and she saw blood dripping from Rimi's smiling mouth. Mina ran downstairs and draped the child's head in kitchen towel. The flow of red subsided and Mina's fear gave way to easy anger. Frowning, scowling all sweaty and hot, Mina shouted 'Why do I have such a stupid child?'

Rimi looked up with her brown eyes and squeezed out a soft, warm smile. Too tense, too creased up inside, Mina continued with her 'idiot, stupid little idiot' just long enough for the tears to kick in. Rimi was soon screaming her head off. Mina was all twisted up inside with nothing to give. She didn't know how long Rimi cried. The wretched sound seemed to consume everything, time, peace and sense. Mina couldn't stop it. Didn't have the energy. Drained and pale she dumped Rimi in the cot and went to bed only getting up when she heard Ravi walk through the front door. He was running now. Running upstairs. The first thing he saw was Rimi, bright pink, cheeks wet with tears stretching her arms out for Daddy.

'What did you do to her?' Ravi was holding Rimi tight in his arms.

'I didn't do anything,' said Mina sitting at her dressing table with her back to Ravi.

'Well how come there is blood on her lip?'

'She ate some glass.'

'What kind of mother are you?' Ravi examined Rimi's swollen lip as she gurgled happily in her Daddy's arms.

'Just shut up.' Mina couldn't keep it together. She was shaking, trying to control her temper; in the end she thumped the bed and kicked the wardrobe. Ravi walked out with Rimi, leaving Mina to simmer. Lying alone on the bed Mina worked herself up into a mini frenzy. 'I'm pregnant, my husband is cheating on me and I'm a shit mother. I should never have married this man. I should never have come to Manchester. I was a bloody fool.'

There was a kick in her stomach that jerked her back to reality. Mina got up. Walked to the bathroom. Opened the glass cabinet door. It was empty apart from some cotton buds, a jar of astral, half a bottle of Paracetamol and a bottle of Sonadine. Mina stretched out a hand and examined the bottle of Sonadine. 'Two tablets to be taken 20 minutes before going to bed, or as directed by your doctor...' The bottle was full. There were at least fifty tablets. She emptied them into her palm and the tablets stared up at her begging to be eaten. She found herself chewing on all 50 tablets one by one. They tasted bitter but it seemed like the right thing to do. Mina quickly felt sleepy and as she reached out for the wall she caught her reflection in the mirror. Looked like she was foaming at the mouth. It was just a little drool. There was another kick in her stomach a little more violent than the last. She stuck her hand down her throat, puked into the toilet and coughed herself into consciousness. Still feeling drowsy she went to bed in a weird sort of stupor. Six hours later, waking up woozy with a splitting headache she thought she was dead but she opened her eyes and seeing Ravi sleeping beside her realised 'I'm alive.' Mina saw a Yellow Pages sitting on the bedside table. Seeing Ravi lying there, all perfect and at peace, she picked up the Yellow Pages and whacked him on the head to purge the pain. Ravi jolted up and almost hit her before quickly restraining himself. He could see the hurt in her eyes. He could see that she was not all there. He pulled the Yellow Pages from her hands and whispered 'Will you please stop all this, I don't love her I love you.' The words assuaged Mina slightly but the pain of that letter still stung.

Mina couldn't seem to get rid of Dimna. She was sitting on a comfy chair in the living room of Mina's brain, looking smug. Mina tried to carry on. She was a mother now with responsibilities. She didn't have time to mope, to shout, to hate, to dwell she was too busy getting on with life, returning library books, going to Asda, tending to roses, wiping Rimi's nose and preparing for baby number two. Months crawled by and Dimna's residue still clung to the cracks of her thoughts and slipped into the holes of her mind. However hard she tried, Mina couldn't forget.

GUNGI BLUES

Bela

Ravi was certain that Bela was a boy when he saw her mass of thick brown curls and her solid, Milky Way thighs. He could not conceal his disappointment when he discovered she was only a girl. She was born 9 March 1972. Ravi walked out the hospital room and sat in the corridor with his head in his arms. He did not hold the newborn child. He did not thank Allah that she was healthy and alive. He did not want to know. Amit Bai sat by Mina's side and, assuming that he was the father, the nurse placed Bela in his arms. Slightly embarrassed, Amit Bai held Bela as she screamed the place down, then he handed her back to Mina. Her face was pale, her eyes sunken, she had been in labour for ten hours and Ravi was sitting outside sulking.

On the way home, Mina cradled her baby in silence and Amit Bai sat with Rimi on his knee, crushed by the tension in the car. Deep inside Mina felt like some kind of genetic failure for being unable to produce that precious son. Once at home, Mina began to mutter

'Why are you so obsessed with boys? What's the big deal?' who cares?'

'I've always wanted a son. Every father wants a son. Don't you want a son Amit Bai?' Amit Bai didn't answer.

'You haven't even looked at her. Why don't you look at her? Go on look at her,' Mina held Bela up in her arms; her head was swaying in circles, her eyes searching wildly.

'Just leave it OK,' Ravi turned to Amit Bai and asked

'Do you want a cup of tea?'

'Cup of tea, I shit on your cup of tea,' said Mina stomping upstairs with Rimi in one arm and Bela in the other. Ravi laughed nervously, shrugged his shoulders and walked into the kitchen.

Mina took the children to the bedroom. She dropped Rimi into the cot and sat on the bed holding Bela in her arms. Bela had hazel eyes, dimpled cheeks and thick lips. Her skin was the colour of Devonshire cream and there were tiny brown curls sprouting from her head. Mina stared at her unwanted children and stared at her tired face in the mirror. She tried to hide her feelings of rejection. She had to keep it together for the children. She had to be a good mother. She had to love her kids and appreciate them. Then she saw Rimi sticking fluff up her nose, yet again, and it was easier to smack than explain. And when Rimi tried to say something to mummy it was easier to say 'shut up' than listen. Rimi avoided Mina preferring to play on her own. In the morning as Ravi prepared to leave for work she gave him a big kiss saying 'hurry Daddy, or you'll be late'. In the evening she waited for Ravi to come home. 'Daddy, Daddy.' She would say when she saw his silhouette through the glass door. Ravi spent time playing with Rimi. He built elaborate castles out of bricks, made up silly stories about dragons and if his imagination ran dry he tickled Rimi until he begged her to stop. He played with her even though he was tired and all he wanted to do was sleep. Sleep temporarily blocked out his worries about money, his job and the new mouth to feed.

On 26 March 1972 the liberation war ensued between East and West Pakistan. It would be nine bloody months until Bangladesh finally achieved victory on 16 December 1972. To the rest of the world the plight of this third world country was small news - not to Ravi, Mina and Amit Bai. They listened to the BBC World Service for any snippet of info. An estimated three million people were killed. The streets of Dhaka were red with blood. Women raped. Babies mutilated. Men tortured. Villages set alight. People abducted. People murdered. These were the kind of horror stories you read about but never imagined happening in your own country. Mina received a letter from Boo Boo describing the moment the Pakistani militia took Boro Kalu away for questioning, 'I was numb with terror' she wrote. 'I watched them take him away and I was left alone with the children. I heard nothing for a week. Then he came back. He'd lost a stone in weight. He looked like a beggar. He showed me his back with deep wounds, all covered in pus. They beat him until he screamed like a baby.' As Mina read the letter, she felt guilty lounging in her cosy sitting room. If she was really honest though she was glad to be in Manchester.

A week after the outbreak of the war Ravi was called into the main office of his bank. His Pakistani boss said 'I'm sorry but I have to let you go.' Ravi didn't have to ask why. He knew it was because he was from the wrong side. Ravi packed his bags and left. Waiting at the bus stop on Wilmslow Road he stared at the scores of glittery shops with flashing pink lights and garish interiors. The new restaurants had naff names like Chilli Cottage and Super Taj and there was an incipient smell of sophistication and affluence lining the curry mile. Then he saw it. A run down unit positioned between a sari shop and restaurant. He approached the window. The place was a shell with bare walls and a flaking lino floor. There was a twinkle in Ravi's eye. A hint of a dream - a grocery store gleaming with plump fresh chillies and bloated watermelons.

That same evening Ravi broke the news to Mina. She was angry that the 'bastards' had sacked him because of the war. It seemed so unfair. Ravi was indifferent because as far as he was concerned they'd have a new grocery shop.

'What do you know about running a business? Why don't you just get another job in a bank,' Mina asked.

Ravi was intransigent and Mina could only sit by and watch as he set about the unit's transformation into a cutting edge grocers. Once he obtained the lease he washed the walls with bleach and built make shift shelves out of old planks. He couldn't afford to buy new lino and couldn't afford staff. Amit Bai offered to help out although he was working as a waiter at night serving poppadums and chutney, steaming naan and chicken tikka. Trying hard not to get the white cuffs of his uniform dirty, trying hard not to sweat, trying to remember his orders and forget that his feet were killing him, Amit Bai worked from four until one in the morning. After the restaurant shut he received the odd left over kebab for his dinner and Amit Bai quickly learnt to slip away to the loo and gorge himself with stolen roshaguli and onion bhajis to sustain him through the night. In between lectures he helped Ravi in the shop. He painted the sign 'Ravi and Sons Grocery store.' Painted it freehand in crimson against navy. He carefully lined the shelves with extra goods like BacoFoil, Libby's fruit cocktail, Sunblest bread, corned beef, Heinz ravioli, garden peas, Jacob's crackers and Rich Tea biscuits. Ravi carefully arranged his lemons, limes, bananas, pineapples, mangoes, aubergines, courgettes, chillies, coriander and other vegetables in neat piles. That first week of trading people didn't come. Customers complained that the veg wasn't fresh. They preferred their local that sold useful extras like Bold washing powder and family sized packs of toilet roll. Ravi was forced to throw out more than he sold after the first day. By the end of the week the shop floor was covered in dirt and bits of green and Ravi was too tired to clean, too tired to think.

A few months after Bela was born Mina fell pregnant again with Ana. She contemplated telling Ravi although she anticipated his response 'Get rid of it. We can't afford it. I don't want another girl.' Like a migrant Ravi drifted in and out the house. He was never around for Mina to break her news. Getting up too early and returning home too late, he made one cursory comment about Mina's expanding waistline saying 'you're getting fat.' Four months later she found a moment to break the good news. This time they didn't fight, they didn't talk about it, because the grocery shop was consuming Ravi, leaving little time to prepare for impending babies.

Mina noticed that Ravi was no longer the lithe man she met four years back. His hair was thinning, his complexion pasty, his belly expanding. Perhaps it was because he insisted on eating two eggs with four pieces of toast oozing with real Cornish butter and smoked a pack of fags per day. Now and then he did some exercise like walk to the corner shop for a paper and only after much nagging did he take up weights. It was while pumping that he felt a stabbing pain in his chest. Sharp and short, it was enough to make an appointment at the hospital a fortnight on Wednesday. A delivery of vegetables came in that day and he cancelled. Ravi didn't bother to make another appointment because the pain dwindled and went away. There were too many chillies to sell and he just couldn't spare the time. Mina started to use vegetable oil instead of Ghee as an incremental step towards a healthier lifestyle. Ravi said that without 'Ghee there's no point eating.' When Mina tentatively suggested that Ravi stopped smoking he replied 'no smoking in the home is like no shitting in the toilet.' Mina gave in and Ravi continued to eat two eggs on buttered toast and fill his lungs with tar.

As Mina soldiered on Bela and Rimi roamed the house like wild animals sniffing out territory to vandalise with their Crayola crayons. They were out of control and Mina was too tired to notice. One Sunday morning Rimi woke up early and dragged Bela out of bed. Ravi and Mina were having a lie in before the arrival of an old friend of Ravi's from Bangladesh. The two sisters crept downstairs to Rimi's favourite corner. Dank and dark under the table, this is where she kept her secret concoctions made up of twig, soil, turmeric and vegetable oil. Rimi had found an exciting new object and she desperately wanted to show Bela. It was an empty Maltesers box, red and shiny almost glistening in the morning sun light. Bela stared blankly at the box and was not impressed. But Rimi had a cunning plan for her beautiful Maltesers box. From the age of two Rimi had developed a nasty habit of playing with dirt like substances. She would mould handfuls of the filthy brown stuff into small balls. Round, brown and very smooth. She bottled her creations in old glass jars for quite some time until one day she got caught. Stupidly, she gave a jar to

Amit Bai as a gift. At first he stared in wonderment at the brown round things floating in a green washing up liquid solution. But then, when he unscrewed the jar, he nearly fainted from the stink. From that day onwards Rimi was officially banned from bottling her balls but the yearning to collect them was innate. Now at last Rimi had found a new home for her brown round friends. Rimi sat and concentrated as she moulded and squeezed. Bela watched her big sis in awe. There they sat, two little people shrouded in white lace tablecloth. Rimi moulded the dirt with real dexterity. Then she paused before carefully placing the three brown balls in the Maltesers box. They looked like delicious, glistening chocolate Maltesers. No one would tell the difference apart from the smell. The sound of heavy footsteps made Rimi and Bela freeze on the spot. In a lightning flash she hid the box behind the table leg and sat quiet and still with Bela by her side. Amit Bai smiled at them, scooped up Bela and guided them into the kitchen for breakfast. Bela kept her soiled fists clenched but Amit Bai didn't notice. As Bela and Rimi ate their Weetabix all they could think about was the Maltesers box.

Mina was busy pouring Domestos down the loo and fiddling with the curtains. The house was transformed from a dusty dump to an immaculate, almost sparkling flash place. Late that afternoon the guest from Bangladesh arrived with a tired face and battered suitcase. His name was Mucki. He was a shiny brown man with a shiny matching dome of a head that he rubbed occasionally with a certain pleasure. He beamed at the two little ones and patted Rimi's head like a dog before picking Bela up. Within ten minutes Bela drooled on his freshly dry cleaned jacket and Bela happily farted on his knee. It was only Rimi who charmed him with a gummy smile. After he had done his bonding Mucki ignored them. When a child is ignored they usually demand more attention. Rimi just couldn't understand why nice Mr Mucki was so hostile now. She decided to offer him a nice home made Malteser to make him warm and friendly once more. Amit Bai and Ravi were too engrossed in conversation to notice Rimi slipping under the table to retrieve her red box. And Mina was too busy perfecting her plough rice to see Rimi creep past. Undetected, Rimi planted the box bang in the middle of Mucki's bed. It wasn't until the evening that he tasted his bedtime treat. When he saw the chocolates he became so overcome with greed that he gorged on them before the smell hit him like a slap in the face and he puked all over the bed.

After the Malteser incident rather than shy away from entertaining, Ravi just couldn't turn anyone away. Meeting people took his mind off the shop. Talking, eating and laughing kept him going. He was too much of a social animal. Mina would complain 'Why do you bring all these people into my house. Who are they?'

'I just met them in the store,' he would reply with a smile and then he returned to his newfound friends leaving Mina to chop the onions.

Mina couldn't understand Ravi's desire to entertain when the grocery store was losing money by the day. To save money Mina used multi-layered cloth nappies with safety pins that ate into soft skin. She washed those cloth nappies with her bare hands because they didn't have a washing machine. A life of domestic toil was so far removed from Mina's cushy life in Pathuakali where she never lifted a finger apart from to turn the pages of her books. Mina recalled how she was the one who excelled at school. She was the one Nanu boasted about. She was the one who, apart from a slight bud bud accent, spoke English perfectly. With her brains and looks she was going to excel and lead a flash life. At least that's what everyone thought. Now her sisters were married to army officers, living off the government and spitting out orders to servants. It was ironic that Mina was the one who ended up washing nappies.

Despite being hard up for cash, Mina saved up for three months to have her bedroom painted a cool shade of green. She painted the walls herself. The colour green made her feel calm and reminded her of home. That same morning the shabby glass door was being re-fitted with a fancy trim. She was going to surprise Ravi with her home improvements. It would cheer him up. Take his mind off the rotten business. In long strokes she painted for three hours only pausing for a cup of tea and a digestive. Eager to finish the job she ran upstairs to find Bela drawing palm trees and boats above the skirting boards. The drawings were really rather good.

'Bela,' Mina screamed.

Bela's body jumped up and she made a final flash of lightning with her blue crayon. Mina banished Bela downstairs where she was happy to watch the man fit glass. Bela blinked dopily at the glass panel. It flashed and sparkled in the light. The man turned his back for a second. Bela only meant to touch it and ended up walking straight through the glass. There was a colossal crash. Mina came hurtling downstairs. The glass man was motionless and Bela sat in the midst of a sea of glass with a tiny drop of blood dripping from her nose. When Ravi came home to find the mess of glass in the hallway he didn't make a fuss. Mina stopped her DIY efforts but she continued to carry four bags of shopping, prepare elaborate meals and dig in the garden. She tried to touch up her make up before Ravi came home, change her outfit and look nice for her husband. She was always striving for perfection.

Ana

One Sunday morning, Mina felt strangely dizzy. She traipsed upstairs for a nap. Half an hour later, she woke up to discover Ana in a bloody mess oozing out her legs. Ana wasn't due for another month but she arrived on 28 April 1973. The mattress was drenched in red and Mina started to wail hysterically. Amit Bai ran in to see a small gooey head sticking out of Mina's open legs. He stood paralysed staring as Mina screamed in pain. Amit Bai ran out and knocked frantically on Miss Redfern's door.

'I'm sorry I'm busy. Why don't you call an ambulance? That's what most people do' she replied coolly.

'But the baby's on its way out,' Amit Bai pleaded.

Miss Redfern didn't want to know and closed the door. Amit Bai cursed her under his breath before trying the Walsh's. He banged on the door with both fists and seeing his distraught face Mrs Walsh came to help. By now Mina was barely conscious and Ana's head was stuck. Mrs Walsh helped to ease out the head and the ambulance men arrived to find there was nothing to be done apart from pat Mrs Walsh on the back. Ravi came home that evening to discover his new daughter staring with big eyes. This time Ravi hid his disappointment put his arm around his wife and checked she was all right. Outwardly Ravi put on a big smile. Played happy father. Took a picture of the three children perfectly posed on the sofa. Rimi was smiling holding Bela in her podgy arms and Bela was giggling so hard that her thick curls wobbled. Ana lay at their feet, staring into the camera with a frown and clenched fist. There was a halo of healthiness in that photo. Everything looked golden. The family was now complete.

For the first week Ana didn't stop crying. Amit Bai tried all kinds of tricks, took her for long walks, tried to pat the child into slumber, sang Bangla songs, and threw Ana up in the air. He tried it all. Ana's crying was loud and unrelenting. It drowned out the silence, upset Rimi, made Bela whimper, killing any moment for reflection. Mina and Ravi sat up all night trying to shut the child up. After three hours sleep, Ravi crawled out of bed at six in the morning, eyes blood shot and face swollen, to open up the shop. Night after night Ana terrorised her parents with incessant screams. Ana swallowed up their attention when Bela needed a cuddle and Rimi wanted to play. Occasionally she gave them relief for half an hour before the sobs churned up her puny body, her face turned pink, her eyes creased up and that sound exploded out Ana's tiny mouth. Mina took her daughter to the doctor. He suggested bathing Ana's head in cool water. It didn't work. Nothing worked for months.

On a bitterly cold January afternoon Ravi came home early from the shop. Mina was out with Bela and Ana. Amit Bai was playing with Rimi in the small-room. Ravi helped himself to something to eat, went to the toilet and chatted with Amit Bai and Rimi before deciding to take a nap on the sofa in the front room. He never usually took a nap but he felt particularly weak and exhausted. At 3.39 in the afternoon he had his first heart attack. Rimi was the one who discovered him laid out like a beached whale, hand hung limply at his side, mouth open releasing a steady stream of dribble. She thought that Daddy was playing a game. She copied Daddy and pretended to be dead too. Then she became bored when Daddy didn't move as she tugged persistently at his hand and climbed all over him, like a cheeky monkey, pulling at his big ears and tweaking his nose.

A fat ambulance nee nawed into Whitebrook Road. People, despite themselves, could not resist a gawp. Amit Bai and Mina shoved all three children in the back of the ambulance and they all squashed together around Ravi, hard and grey like a concrete slab. He looked dead already. Mina just stared at her husband in disbelief. It must be scary when one so young is hanging precariously in the balance of life and death and there's absolutely nothing you can do but pray to the clouds, the sun, Allah, God, Buddah, anything and anybody, that in thirty seconds the man laying there before you will laugh in your face and break out in deep song. Instead Ravi lay, looking more green than grey now with his lids slightly open showing the whites of his eyeballs' like an alien from Star Trek. Rimi and Bela didn't fathom the gravity of the situation. Bela was too busy playing with things she shouldn't have and unzipping curious white bags containing plastic tubes. Rimi just thought that Daddy had a bug up his nose; that he would be better soon; and that she would ride his back later that evening round and round the onyx table until she became dizzy and fell off with a soft thud. Amit Bai could not bear to look his best friend in the eye and instead peered out the window at the sun set. Pastel lemons and tufts of orange curled happily in that swirling sky. Amit Bai was transfixed and the painting in the sky soothed his aching soul for a minute or two until the colours were erased with dirty grey sheets of cloud.

They pulled up outside St Mary's hospital where Rimi and Bela were born. St Mary's had been good to Mina, delivering her children healthy and ripe. Ravi was in healing hands there. They rushed him away in a whirlwind of white flapping coats and he was gone. Mina, Amit Bai and the kids were left standing like fools in the middle of the hospital floor. Ana was screaming the place down, Rimi was trying to escape, and Bela had run off with a little old lady in a zimmer frame. Mina didn't seem to care. She just stood and stared as if stuck in time, with her feet firmly Bostik glued to the floor, as Amit Bai ran after Bela with Ana hanging from his arms and Rimi running by his side. A chubby nurse with a soft face guided them to some shiny, grey plastic chairs. Waiting and waiting. Three hours trickled by in ten. The doctors and nurses stood whispering in a corner before approaching Mina. She expected the worst. Rimi and Bela were skidding down the long polished corridors in their socks like a pair of drug-crazed loonies. Mina let them scream and shout, while Ana lay limply on her lap bawling her eyes out. After half an hour of banshee type screaming, a nurse quietly told Bela and Rimi to put their shoes back on and settle down before suggesting to Mina that Ana might be hungry. Like a zombie she stuck a bottle in Ana's mouth and that temporarily shut her up. Then a tall doctor in a gleaming white coat walked towards Mina and whispered something in her ear. The fleeting relaxation of Mina's face faded. Her skin became wrinkled up in a state of anxiety. Amit Bai sat in silence looking down at his feet knowing that words were futile.

Hours later Rimi and Bela lay sprawled out on plastic chairs asleep. Ana was still whimpering refusing nastily to give Mina any relief. In desperation Amit Bai picked Ana up and as he paced back and forth he patted her hard on the back beating the baby into a numb sleep. There was peace at last. A quiet moment where Mina could order the chaos that whirred in her head.

A sharp silence filled the corridor now, the fluorescent light bounced off the polished floor and glared in their faces giving everyone a sickly green pallor. The only sound was snuffled breathing and the smacking of lips. Seeing the children entangled messily on the uncomfortable plastic chairs, a concerned nurse suggested that everyone go home and get some sleep. Mina refused at first but after, twenty minutes of soft, subtle persuasion, she relented. Exhausted, the bags under Mina's eyes seemed to pull her face down towards the polished floor. As Mina and Amit Bai bundled the children all together into a lumpy heap a crazy commotion suddenly broke out and the sound of running feet echoed in the corridors. Doctors with flapping white coats skidded into the room where Ravi lay with a plastic tube stuck up his nose on his flat white bed in his clean white room. Mina froze and she dropped Ana on the floor.

Ravi had a second fatal heart attack and died at 4.09 am, 14 January 1974. He was thirty-four years old. Mina was twenty-five, Rimi was three, Bela was one and a half and Ana was eight months old.

Mina was asleep, the mumblings had ceased and Ana sat and watched the quiver of her brow as she snored slightly. Widowed at twenty five years old with three young kids. Ana tried to imagine her mother's grief. There is a famous painting by Picasso of the 'Weeping Woman.' The painting that art critics say conveys human despair in its most acute form. But that painting failed to convey Mina's grief. Mina still saw Ravi in her dreams. He visited her every night. Perhaps he was watching over her now and they were having a conversation. Ana was ambivalent about her father with his movie star looks, oozing charm and European girlfriends. He wanted all his children aborted. He was obsessed with boys and never wanted girls. If Mina had listened to him Ana wouldn't be standing as an adult looking over her mother now. That label of accidental birth haunted every one of her sisters. Ana lay on the bed next to her mother and staring up at the ceiling thought about the past. Her childhood in 6 Whitebrook Road, growing up with her sisters and Mina's struggle to overcome the loss of Ravi and live a new life.

GUNGI BLUES

New Life

When the doctor told Mina that her husband was dead she didn't believe him. How could Ravi be dead? He'd barely lived. Barely enjoyed the children. Barely tasted life. Somehow, it didn't seem right. Ravi was going to walk through that door, tired and hungry, and Mina was going to find him in the living room lighting up a cigarette. She only found stubbed out cigarette ends in the ashtray. Alone in her bed, a bed that seemed huge and lonely for one, Mina cried and cried. Loud, hefty sobs that left her face aching. In the daytime Mina roamed the house looking slightly lost, her eyes had a permanent glazed watery look about them. She longed for night. That was when she could sleep and live life through her dreams. That was when Mina saw Ravi's face. Smiling. Singing. Laughing. Sure, they'd argued, she'd shouted, nagged and whinged but that didn't matter, they were happy, in a funny sort of way.

With no job, three kids, a mortgage, too many plants, a house filled with shadows and a ten tonne brick of grief hanging around her neck, a metaphorical nuclear bomb suddenly obliterated Mina's world. The weight fell off Mina's cheeks and her squidge and plumpness quickly shrank. Two stones lighter, battered and weak, she was a widow, with nothing in her handbag apart from a few pounds in her purse. Soon she'd be on housing benefit. What choice did she have? There looked like there was no future in Manchester. Nana called everyday, leaving the same message: ‘hello, it’s Daddy. Come home. Thank you. Goodbye.’ In Bangladesh, as a widow with three kids, the only future was one of pity. She was better off in England, she thought. At night as her head hit the pillow and the left-hand side of the bed remained cold she thought she’d be better off dead.

Mina was often sleeping in the early afternoon. She didn’t want to talk, to play or read so the children turned to Amit Bai. Listening to them squabble and laugh was some comfort. It took his mind off things. Amit Bai was twenty-seven now, he’d just graduated. He was more than satisfied with his third class degree. As he said ‘a degree is a degree’ and he wasn’t the type of person to brood. His third class degree didn’t stop the triple job offers coming in either. He accepted a position at Norweb as a computer operator. Several weeks before Ravi died, Amit Bai broke the good news of his new job to Ravi and they hugged a tight bear hug with joy. They were going to celebrate with a party the following week. Amit Bai felt his future was bright; he never did get to celebrate with Ravi, instead they had a simple meal of dhal, rice, and mango pickle. They finished off their meal, belched and picked their teeth before going to bed. Amit Bai lay in bed thinking of his best friend. In twelve hours life seemed finished. It didn’t make sense that a thirty-four year old man with a wife and three children was suddenly dead. What were they supposed to do now? The reality of the situation was so awesome it was difficult to swallow and it transformed itself into a huge lump that stuck in his throat before transmuting into tears. Amit Bai cried that night. He cried for Ravi to come home.

There was no quiet period to mourn. A steady stream of unfamiliar faces flooded the house. Poured out their condolences, dished out an obligatory spoonful of pity and expected a nice dinner afterwards. Mina fed them with a smile; listened to anecdotes about Ravi, into the small hours of the morning, until finally showing the last guest out. She waved goodbye, shut the door and was finally, left alone with the comfort of her grief. After a month the same faces came sniffing with pseudo smiles and cheap offerings of stale Viennese Truffles. They were all sniffing for a whiff of Mina. She was beautiful. A good cook. Very fertile with a brain too. And then there were the three children. People used to stop in the street and stare at their creamy complexions admiring them like three exotic species in Chester zoo. Bela's hazel eyes and thick and shiny long brown curls. Ana's bright cow eyes, fair skin and fine brown hair. And Rimi, glowing with a radiance that comes from eating three Weetabix each morning. But there was something shifty about these men. Maybe it was their onion smelling armpits and rough skin. Or maybe it was their fawning ways and wandering eyes. Although Mina was always polite declining their offers with grace, inside it made her sick to hear their sugary words knowing that her bed was still warm with the memory of her dead husband.

Two months after Ravi's death Ana started to crawl into Amit Bai's bed at night and rested her head against his dome of a belly. Soon she was calling him 'Daddy,' Ana didn't know any better and Amit Bai didn't object. Bela copied Ana but Rimi still called him Amit Bai. At three years old the memory of Ravi was as strong as a purple ink stain on the carpet. One minute she had been playing with her Daddy, the next thing he was in hospital with a bug up his nose and then he was gone.

Although Rimi saw his face and heard his voice in her sleep, she didn't talk about him. She appeared outwardly normal and never once asked 'Where's Daddy?'

Ravi's body was flown back to Bangladesh to be buried in Dhaka. Afterwards Mina lamented to herself 'I should have shown Rimi his dead body, I should have let her say good bye to Daddy.'

Mina never told Rimi that Ravi was dead and playing with the angels in heaven. She wasn't ready to explain mortality to a four-year old. The children were young. Mina was a baby herself in many ways. It was better to carry on as normal.

1975, a year after Ravi's death, Mina and Amit Bai married. They were all living under the same roof, Ana was calling Amit Bai Daddy, men were coming round for no reason, people were starting to talk and marriage seemed like the ultimate panacea. There were no photographs of a smiling newly wed couple. No red saris, henna or toothpaste dotted decoratively on cheeks. No big wedding party where people dished out the food from buckets. There was no pomp and glitter, no guests, no tears, no laughter.

Leaving the children with Mrs Walsh, Amit Bai and Mina arrived at the registry office on a rainy Manchester morning. Mina's face looked glum. Amit Bai sober. They arrived dressed formally, Mina in a plain blue sari and Amit Bai in his only suit, and waited their turn in the corridor. The couple sitting beside them had splashed out on white lilies. They chatted with one another and Amit Bai couldn't help over hearing about their honeymoon planned in Rome. Mina and Amit Bai were finally called up and directed to a grand room with walls covered in portraits of bald stately figures. They repeated their vows, exchanged rings and did not kiss. They signed the book and two strangers dragged in from the street witnessed the union before Amit Bai and Mina returned to 6 Whitebrook Road on the bus to make rice for the kids.

When Amit Bai broke the news to his folks back in Barisal his mother said

'She's a widow with three kids. You have a degree, a job, a future.'

'It's my business,' replied Amit Bai calmly.

Perhaps he married Mina out of duty to his best friend. Maybe he thought he was getting a good deal. Mina was beautiful, she had three pretty kids and she was the loyal type. If Mina was honest with herself she never found Amit Bai attractive with his Roman nose and pitted cheeks. Still they got on, and could talk about Ravi late into the night without growing bored.

A month into the marriage depression hung over Mina like persistent night. Guilt that she married Amit Bai so soon after Ravi's death; guilt that she was neglecting her three children; and guilt that Amit Bai had to share the burden. Mina visited her GP, saying 'I can't cope, I'd rather be dead'.

In response the GP dished out a colourful cocktail of anti-depressants.

The tablets left Mina drowsy; half the time she forgot where she left them. Usually they sat safely in the bathroom cabinet; occasionally she left them by the bed, where Bela often played with dirty socks and shoes. One quiet Saturday afternoon, Bela discovered the brown bottle that rattled beautifully if shaken and managed to ply it open with her teeth. She poured the whole lot out and made daisy patterns on the carpet. Bela only tried a handful to see if they tasted any good – she ended up knocked out. One hour later Amit Bai went upstairs in search of his false teeth. He usually kept them on the bedside table in a mug. Just as he was putting them in his mouth he saw Bela's foot resting by the empty pill bottle. Amit Bai dropped his teeth and dragged Bela's body from under the bed. No amount of shaking brought the life back to her floppy limbs. Sticking his finger down Bela's throat, Amit Bai forced her to puke. After a few seconds she spluttered and coughed out the pills. Apart from looking slightly green, she was alive. There was no brain damage or anything. When Mina found out, she bought Bela a Mr Silly jigsaw puzzle and a bottle of Lucozade as some kind of compensation for her maternal neglect.

Mina's second flirtation with death changed her. She was freshly married. She'd been given a new start, a chance to re-evaluate her life. She already had a Chemistry degree from Dhaka University and after Ana was born she enrolled for an MSc in Environmental Science at Manchester University. Ravi died and she dropped out before she'd really begun. It didn't matter because she knew damn well that she was clever enough to get a proper job, she didn't want to be on benefit all her life and she couldn't wallow forever. Amit Bai was earning a paltry sixteen pounds a week and it just wasn't enough. With all three children at nursery Mina started to scour the papers for jobs. She saw a small ad in the Manchester Evening News for a cleaning job. The pay was poor but it was a job. Mina called up and arranged an interview. She had never been for a job interview in her life. On the day of her interview, Mina arrived to find a room packed with people all going for the same job. People ranged from scruffy students to ladies wearing slippers with curlers in their hair and fags hanging from their lips'. Mina looked like a Bombay movie star in her red silk sari. After two hours, a short man with two days stubble spread across his face, called out her name. The interview room was sparsely furnished with a brown carpet, a cheap plywood table, two plastic chairs and the air was grey with cigarette smoke. The man started to bombard Mina with complex cleaning questions and she sat dumb. Then she smiled sweetly at the man saying

'I have a Chemistry degree from Dhaka University and I got into Manchester University to do an MSc in Environmental Science. I can speak Hindi, Urdu, Bengali, and English of course, and I can read Arabic. I learn quickly too and ... '

The man stared at Mina, started to itch his head in irritation, and cutting her off in mid sentence said

'I'll let you know, send the next person in on your way out.'

She didn't get the job.

Feeling rather useless, Mina was depressed for several days afterwards. All she needed was the right advice and a gentle push. After wracking her brains she realised that the person who she should really talk to was Mr Allaudin. An old friend of Ravi's, Mr Allaudin was an effervescent man with a permanent smile on his face and a creamy rough voice. Mina called him up and Mr Allaudin invited Mina over to his house for a chat.

Mr Allaudin seemed to collect degrees for a hobby. In total he had two BSc's, two MSc's and two PhD's, one from Oxford and the other from Harvard. His tramp like appearance disguised his shiny brain. He drove an old, dented mini. The original colour had long since flaked away. He always wore the same crumpled grey suit. Fraying at the edges and blotted with crusty food stains, he didn't seem to notice. Mr Allaudin's face was shiny and the foul stench of sweat lingered long after he left a room. Ravi had seen genuine warmth in his smile, vitality in his eyes, a big heart and a great mind. Others could not tolerate his odorous and filthy appearance and shunned him but Mr Allaudin didn't care.

On his way home Mr Allaudin saw Mina standing at the bus stop in the pelting rain. Big globs of water rolled down her cheeks, her toes were drowning in puddles, her silk sari stuck to her like a second skin and she resembled a melting green lollipop. Mr Allaudin swerved onto the pavement and Mina jumped back. He rolled down the window, smiled a yellow stained grin, and said 'Get in Babi, I'll give you a ride.'

Mina obliged and as soon as she closed the door the smell hit her with a pinch. And when he turned to talk she tried to hold her breath as the stench of rotting gums stuck in her nose. Mr Allaudin talked endlessly, reassuring Mina, 'don't worry Babi; you'll have no problem getting a job. No problem at all.'

Mr Allaudin turned into a street lined with dilapidated houses, stopped with a sudden jerk, and reversed with a bang into his driveway. The grass in his garden was jungle high and the house was elegantly peeling. As they entered the house, Mina tried to conceal her shock. Dirty with neglect, the walls were stained, the pattern on the carpet was barely visible and it felt sticky under foot. Mr Allaudin told Mina to feel right at home. He started to make a brew but deciding that tea was not good enough for his guest, he insisted 'I'll make you a delicious drink Babi. Just wait here please.'

Off he scurried into the garden towards a half dead blackberry bush. He enthusiastically started plucking handfuls of dried up berries, ran into the kitchen, dropped half of them on to the floor and stuffed the rest in a cup plucked straight from the sink. There was a carton of milk by the windowsill and he poured it into the cup. Squashing the blackberries into a pulp he added it to the milk and stirred vigorously. Mr Allaudin was so pleased with his fruity cocktail he could not stop grinning. Mina did not want to hurt his feelings after he had gone to so much trouble but couldn't help herself 'I'm sorry, I don't feel too well, could I have a cup of tea instead?' At least tea was made with boiling water she thought.

'Are you sure Babi. It's really delicious' Said Mr Allaudin downing his concoction in one go.

They finally sat down on sticky sofas and Mr Allaudin started going on about his wife. 'She's a pain. Always nagging me. Always saying why can't you earn more money? Why do you drive that crappy mini? Why don't you buy a new suit? She's obsessed with money. It's a disease you know. Anyway she lives in the other house with the kids now. Babi I do miss my kids. Don't know what nonsense she's spitting at them but at least I can write without her nagging and I can read without getting yelled at.' He sighed before his eyes perked up. 'Oh Babi, I'm reading this new book. It's absolutely tremendous. Really tremendous' Mr Allaudin caressed the cover before passing it to Mina.

As Mina examined the book, the sepia hand made paper and the marbled shine of the front, she recalled her chance meeting with Mrs Allaudin at the checkout in Asda some months back.

'How's the grocery business? Heard it's not doing very well. Pity Ravi lost his job. What are you going to do now? Go on benefit.'

These were Mrs Allaudin's first words to her and as she babbled on Mina observed her mean mouth. After a few minutes Mrs Allaudin's high nasal voice gave her a headache. As she ranted on Mina could only stand and listen.

'At least your husband's trying. My husband's useless. The house is falling apart, we have no money and he doesn't do anything apart from write. That stupid man could earn so much but all he cares about are books. Never mind what I want.'

On the day of her marriage Mrs Allaudin erroneously believed her husband's brain would bring them BMW's and a plush house with a double garage not a dirty shack with weeds. Now she couldn't look him in the eye because he made her sick. Mr Allaudin was a failure with stupid letters after his name and not a penny in the bank and when they had sex although Mr Allaudin really tried hard to be a passionate lover, his wife closed her eyes and prayed that Allah would whisk her away into the arms of a Bollywood hunk.

Another hour slipped by and at last Mr Allaudin suddenly remembered the purpose of the visit. 'Oh Babi, I'm sorry we're supposed to talk about jobs. Listen there's something going at the High Court. Interpreters are badly needed. It pays well at fourteen pounds an hour. Here's a pen. Call this number, ask for Russell and mention my name. Call on Tuesday after I've sent a letter of recommendation. Don't you worry Babi, everything will be just fine.'

'Thank you,' Mina gushed.

'It's my pleasure.' Mr Allaudin paused before softening his voice.

'How are you Babi? It must be hard without Ravi. I miss him badly.'

Mina smiled, 'I'm fine' she said as her eyes automatically welled with tears.

.

The next day Mina called up and arranged an interview. The basic requirement was fluency in English and Bangla. She performed a simple test and got the job. Mina was so ecstatic she wept.

A few weeks later Mina heard that Mr Allaudin had suffered an apoplectic stroke and was bedridden. She wondered if anyone visited him, his wife or children perhaps? Nobody did visit him, not even Mina at first. She wanted to but she was afraid of what she might see. Mr Allaudin lay in bed for weeks, unable to move. Once a fortnight a home help came to wash him, clean the house and give him some soup. His skin was congealing into the sheets, his body limp but his brain remained alert and hungry for words. Unable to speak he whimpered and grunted. It was a cry for books. That's all he wanted. Mina eventually did visit to thank him. He lay in his bed like a deformed vegetable. She could see he was happy to see her. She sat and read from a journal for an hour or so and he went to sleep content that night.

When Mina received her first pay cheque she felt euphoric. Staring at the five pound notes stuffed in a brown envelope Mina couldn't stop smiling. The first thing she did was to blow twenty pounds on two saris from a cheap shop in Rusholme. She wanted to look nice for work. Each morning she tied her hair up in a chic Hepburn bun and flashed a mouth of bright red lipstick. When the CID officers first saw her walk through the door their eyes perked up. Mina thought that they were all very 'dashing' in their freshly pressed uniforms and shiny shoes. When one officer propositioned her 'Oi Min, Fancy goin' out one evening for a drink' Mina bluntly told him about her 'three kids and their new dad'. The officer quickly lost interest and the other men soon ignored her after that.

Mina's main focus was work. She translated all the legal terminology into Bangla even though she didn't have to. She worked harder than her white counterparts staying late and doing extra hours when the office was empty. During meetings she observed her colleagues, arms neatly folded, eyes focused. She tried to emulate them, suppressing the desire to scratch her armpit and sniff it in public. On Mina's second day at work her boss, Keith remarked

'Pooh what's that smell?'

Mina realised it was her garlic stinking hands and she promptly camouflaged the odour with a healthy spray of Estee Lauder perfume in the ladies toilets.

Very quickly she learnt to dampen the bud bud in her accent. Practised saying fruit instead of prut and zoo instead of joo. She became a hybrid; it was the only way to survive.

Mina knew they all thought she was a docile, dopey thing. She felt their eyes watching her shuffle to the photocopying machine. She made their coffee and stapled copies of useless reports. She did it all with a smile. After a while Mina became restless with the irregular hours. She was sick of waiting for the phone to ring and sick of waiting on Keith and Sarah. It became an ordeal to get out of bed each morning. 'I want a salary with a pension' Mina thought. For months she believed it was only a matter of time before she got her teeth into a proper job. She realised the futility of dreaming about it; Mina needed to sort her life out.

Some weeks later Mina saw an advertisement in the Manchester Evening News. The ad was so tiny that she had to use a magnifying glass to read the print. It read 'Job Creation Scheme designed to help local people work in the heart of Oldham's community.' Working in the community was fine but the pay was rubbish and where was Oldham? Nevertheless, Mina felt compelled to circle the ad with a fat red lumocolour pen and dropped it in a bag along with all the other life-changing jobs. The High Court had not called Mina for a whole week and she was lying idle, staring at the ceiling, twiddling her thumbs and picking her feet. She decided to enquire about the Job Creation Scheme.

One phone call later she lined herself up with an interview. Tuesday came and Mina contemplated pulling out and staying in bed after discovering that Oldham was miles away. She forced herself to get dressed, ate half a bowl of Frosties and left for the bus stop. It was not too late for Mina to turn back, sit by the phone and wait for it to ring but the very prospect filled her with a certain dread. Despite herself she boarded several buses and frowned all the way. When she reached her stop she was already fifteen minutes late for her interview. She looked in her purse. There was not enough money for a cab and barely enough for her bus fare home. She scoured her A-Z for the little side street. After half an hour of roaming around and asking unhelpful strangers on the street for directions Mina came across a shabby, run down building on a deserted back street. It looked like a brothel. She checked the address; this was the place. She was one hour late and Mina wondered if she'd already blown it. If she was really honest she was reluctant to go in until she saw a smiling lady, wearing a cream shirt and pleated skirt. Drawn in by the lady's big smile Mina timidly followed her up a narrow flight that led to a dingy corridor. On entering the interview room, Mina was greeted by a panel of beaming people.

'Please come in and sit down. Would you like a Bourbon Biscuit?' said the woman with the big smile

Mina was a little surprised but took a biscuit all the same.

'Can I take your coat?' asked a man in a woolly jumper with bobbly bits hanging from the cuffs.

Feeling her armpits dripping with sweat Mina shook her head and said in a soft polite voice 'no thank you. I'll keep it on. It's a bit cold isn't it?'

The man turned the fan heater under the table on full blast.

'Is that better?' he asked.

The man returned to his seat and began to sift through his notes.

'Can you tell me a little about your background before we start?'

'Well I did Matrix in 1963 and I did intercourse in 1965.'

The man looked a little shocked and intervened.

'You mean intermediate.'

'Yes that's what I said,' replied Mina not realising the slip.

The man couldn't help smiling. His expression changed to one of concern and he said in a gentle voice

'It says here in my notes that you were very recently widowed.'

The panel all looked very sorry and shook their heads in a spontaneous display of sympathy.

'That's right,' Mina replied firmly.

'Now I know it's a sensitive point and if you don't want to talk about it that's OK'

Thinking that it was really none of their business Mina just nodded.

'I mean it really is very tragic isn't? How old was your husband, if you don't mind me asking?'

'Thirty-four.'

'And you are, how old?'

'Twenty-five.'

'Yes that really must be quite terrible.'

Mina wasn't laughing.

'It must be hard bringing up three children all on your own' added the woman with the big smile.

GUNGI BLUES

'You know you shouldn't feel depressed about the situation. In fact if I were in your shoes I would feel extremely proud. I mean bringing up three children, that's a terrific achievement you know. It really is.'

Mina listened quietly as the panellists continued to commend her fortitude.

After another twenty minutes of probing personal questions about coping with widowhood interspersed with the odd mandatory question about 'Experience' and 'Education' the panel convened for an intense period of deliberation that lasted two minutes before the man announced 'we've decided to offer you the job. You have everything we are looking for. The decision was quite unanimous. We'll send you a formal offer in the post with all the contractual details. We don't usually tell candidates on the spot but we've made an exception in your case. I mean you're exactly the sort of person we're looking for.'

Mina didn't try and conceal her disappointment. All she could think about was the dramatic cut in pay if she accepted the position.

The man noticed Mina's sulky face and asked 'Well aren't you happy then?'

Mina nodded before saying quite bluntly 'I'll only take this job if I can come in to work at 10.30. I can not make it at 9 because I have three kids to drop off at nursery and then it will take me another hour, depending on the traffic, to get into work.'

The man was very accommodating. The terms and conditions arrived in the post, Mina signed the contract and started her new job on Monday. The first week wasn't easy for her. With Amit Bai working the night shift he didn't get home until six and then he went straight to bed. Mina was the one who woke up at seven. She gave the children breakfast, plaited their hair, and dumped them at nursery, before embarking on an epic journey to Oldham every morning.

With two steady incomes and Rimi turning four, Mina and Amit Bai started to think about schools. In Fallowfield the local comprehensive was Whalley Range. The school kids there wore dirty brown blazers and bright yellow shirts. Mina watched them board the bus and listened to their slang: 'Are you startin'. Are yer? I'll twat yer I will. I will if yer don't shut it.' With their hard Mancunian accents, their gelled back hair and their rolled up skirts, they didn't seem like schoolgirls. They were the kind of girls who would chew you up and spit you out like gum.

Mina was sitting on the bus to Chorlton-Cum-Hardy on a Saturday afternoon when she spotted sprightly boys in tiny shorts and girls in pleated skirts running around in a playground. Carrying Ana in one arm, the pram in the other, with Bela trailing two steps behind, Mina got off at the next stop to investigate.

GUNGI BLUES

Planted in between two elegant Conifers was a large black sign. It read Amberleigh Preparatory School for girls and boys aged four-eleven. The school resembled a big old house with a front garden lined with delicate pink rose bushes. The children looked immaculate in their blue bobbled berets, cute red blazers and stripy blue ties. Mina looked down at Bela and Ana squashed next to each another in a pram designed for one. The pram was knackered, Bela's bib was stained and Ana was wearing an oversized sweater. Mina looked out at the other children and for a moment she saw her three children standing in that playground, all red and shiny, grinning hand in hand. Scribbling down the phone number of the school on her bus ticket, she stuck it in her purse.

After an hour of staring at the bland displays in shop windows Mina caught the bus home. The image of those little school children in their dapper uniforms and shiny hair stuck in her memory and she almost missed her stop. Pushing her pram down a small leafy sidewalk she saw Rimi swinging like a monkey from a climbing frame. Kids sat on the grass building multi-coloured structures out of bricks, sketching lollipop trees on scraps of paper and nursery teachers hovered in the background. It was a place full of wide-open greenery, splendid old trees and scores of kids, running wild and free. Mina called for Rimi and she ran towards her with the obedience of a well-trained dog. A fresh-faced nursery teacher, with strands of hair obscuring her face, came running towards Mina with Rimi's coat. Mina almost didn't want to leave.

Faced with the noise and dirt of the busy main road, a line of tension severed Mina's forehead in two. 'Hold my hand,' she shouted at Rimi as she struggled to push the pram over the curb.

Once they reached home Mina dumped the three kids in the living room and sat Ana on her knee. She started to pat her back. 'There's a good girl. Go on, do a big burp for mummy.' She cooed.

Ana didn't let out a sound. Mina put her down next to Bela who was just sitting, body floppy with blank eyes. Ana crawled up to her big sister; Rimi's black shiny hair was so enticing, Ana pulled at it hard and Rimi gently pushed her sister's hand away. Ana pulled again until Rimi toppled over, then she climbed onto her face, flattening her chubby cheeks with her foot. Bela looked on dopily and then threw her body onto Rimi's stomach. Mina listened to Rimi's muted cries for help but she didn't intervene. Mina walked into the hallway and made a call instead.

'Hello is that Amberleigh?'

'Yes, this is Amberleigh Preparatory School' was the deep voiced reply.

GUNGI BLUES

'My daughter is very restless. I don't think she is getting enough stimulation. You do take four-year olds don't you?'

The deep voiced man answered.

'Yes we do but your daughter will have to take an entry exam first and then we'll just wait and see.'

'An exam but she's only four,' exclaimed Mina.

'All the children at Amberleigh have to take an exam. How's next Tuesday after school?'

'It should be fine. My name's Mina and what's yours please?' she asked.

'Mr Hayden.'

The following Tuesday Mina accompanied Rimi to Amberleigh. Wearing a bright flower print dress, frilly ankle socks, patent leather shoes with her hair tied up in two bunches, Rimi looked dressed for a party. Standing in the middle of the deserted playground was a tall plank of a man with a bald egghead. Tufts of red hair exploded out his nose and his high arched brow made his expression permanently exclamatory. Fearful of the fire spurting out his nostrils Rimi edged towards the silky walls of Mina's sari. Greeting Mina with a firm handshake Mr Hayden politely asked her to wait inside and relax with a glass of orange squash and a ginger biscuit.

Squatting down Mr Hayden looked Rimi in the eye. She stared at his huge face, his pale blue eyes, his hooked nose, dry lips and his red hair. Delving deep into his jacket pocket, Mr Hayden produced a note pad and a red felt tip pen. After a long pause he said seriously ‘Do you like drawing?’ Rimi nodded.

'Good because I would like you to draw a picture of me.' Mr Hayden handed her the pen and note pad.

Tentatively, Rimi produced a shaky square, an oblong head, two dots for eyes, two squiggles for eyebrows and a slash of a mouth.

'What are those?' asked Mr Hayden pointing at the lines.

'It's the fire coming out your nose and ears.'

'Very good. Now do you like maths?' he said clapping his hands together.

Rimi nodded.

'What's 4 plus 2.'

'6' whispered Rimi automatically.

'Very good. I think you would do very well here Rimi.'

GUNGI BLUES

Rimi smiled shyly and Mr Hayden patted her on the head.

Amit Bai picked up Rimi from school everyday. Rimi would wait by the gates in the playground, neatly buttoned up with her beret on straight and her white socks pulled up. Mr Hayden was never far away, towering over his kiddies like a stone statue.

'Hello,' said Mr Hayden shaking Amit Bai's hand as he approached Rimi.

'You should be proud of Rimi, she's top of her class,' said Mr Hayden beaming at Amit Bai.

'That's very good. Do you think she'll get into Oxford?' said Amit Bai putting his hand on Rimi's shoulder.

'It's too early to tell? She's only four' said Mr Hayden.

Amit Bai waved at Mr Hayden as he walked out the gates holding Rimi's hand.

Sitting on the bus home, Rimi saw two kids eating bon bons from a paper bag, and another was stuffing his mouth with prawn cocktail Skips, the ones that melt on the tongue if you suck them hard. Rimi watched the kids pop yellow bon bons like crisps; she was transfixed until Amit Bai diverted her attention with a question.

‘Rimi, what’s 17 - 9?’

‘Don't know Daddy.’

‘Come on Rimi, think.’

‘Errm seven.’

‘No’ Amit Bai said smacking her head.

‘Think Rimi.’

Rubbing her head Rimi said ‘Eleven Daddy.’

‘That’s right, you can watch Blue Peter if you tell me what 20 - 3 is.’ Rimi frowned with concentration trying to work out the sum as Skips and Bon bons flashed before her.

‘Come on Rimi, hurry up.’ Closing her eyes, Rimi answered

‘Seventeen Daddy. Is that right?’

‘Good girl.’ Amit Bai said squeezing Rimi’s knee.

Rimi quickly learnt the rudiments of Pavlovian conditioning: good behaviour was reinforced with rewards, perhaps a smile, and a gentle rub of the head or an extra sweetie. Errors punished with slaps, no Blue Peter or worse, no Starsky and Hutch.

GUNGI BLUES

At school Rimi sat at her desk and usually finished her work before the others. Rimi didn't chat when Mrs Gilbert turned her back; she only opened her mouth to answer questions. Mrs Gilbert, a scary looking lady with pointy green glasses who clearly dyed her hair red, rewarded excellence with booming gusto. 'Well done Rimi.' 'Right again Rimi.' 'Two gold stars for you Rimi.'

Clever kids usually get beaten up for being swots. Rimi rarely did, perhaps because her expression remained neutral however gushing the praise. She avoided smug smiles, boasting or flashing her gold stars under the noses of her classmates. She just got on with her work. Neatly wrote out her tables, did her sums, copied out passages about John and Jane hopping down the lane. She made extra sure that the bottoms' of her letters sat neatly in her lined textbook. She crossed out using a single line, never scribbled. And she did it all with a robotic efficiency. She didn't have to be warned a second time; didn't need the sting of the ruler.

One morning Mrs Gilbert said 'Stand up Rimi and read your poem to the rest of the class. Now listen carefully everybody. Go on Rimi.' Coaxed Mrs Gilbert with a smile.

Rimi stood up in front of a sea of bored faces and twiddling thumbs. Her paper began to shake in her sweaty palms. Taking a deep breath, she swallowed her fear and read:

Sanchita Islam

The scent of the lilac spread on a sheet
A violet veil on the queen of night
Violet, violet makes me all comfortable and warm
The night sky is smooth and rare
Nobody is to compare with violet but me

Rimi pronounced each word with considered precision. A couple of kids smirked in class but Rimi's face didn't flicker with embarrassment. She just said 'Thank You' and sat down.

At home Rimi liked to sit under her bed and read by torchlight. Her eyes, bespectacled in pink plastic NHS frames, skimmed over the words. The faster she read the greater her satisfaction. Spending most of her time in her room Rimi only ever came downstairs to eat or watch a bit of telly. It was quiet under the bed. There she could write poems, read comics or suck on her secret stash of sweets. Sometimes Amit Bai would come in for a rant

'Rimi you have to work hard. You have to be number one. Number two, number three, number four is not good enough.'

Rimi would listen quietly. It was simpler that way. There was no point trying to argue. It was better to let Amit Bai go on then he would tire and slip away. On one occasion though, Rimi interrupted his 'you have to be number one speech.' She didn't feel like it that day so she pulled out the folded piece of paper sitting in her pocket and asked

GUNGI BLUES

'Daddy do you want to read my poem?'

Amit Bai slowly mumbled the words on the page

Sadness is taking over me, won't let my happiness be
Sadness is pushing me down, won't let me be free
I'm just a small bee
Happiness won't take my hand,
Everything is different
I'm on a different land
Happiness won't go through the hall
I'm just a small mole
You're greater than me
You're bigger
You're greater and larger than me
I'm smaller than you.

'Very good now put it away and learn your seven times tables then you can watch telly.' Said Amit Bai finishing his tea.

It was Saturday morning and Rimi was sitting at the kitchen table, writing a shopping list in perfect hand. Milk, eggs, bread, Sugar Puffs. Mina was curled up in her double bed with Bela on one side and Ana on the other. Rimi tip toed into the bedroom opened Mina's handbag and took some money from her purse. Just enough. She dragged a chair from the kitchen, climbed up to open the front door and walked to the shop down the road. The shopping bag Rimi carried under her arm was half her size. Standing on the corner was the supermarket. 'Buy one can of Spaghetti Hoops and get one Free' was splashed on the glass windows. Rimi pushed open the door with some difficulty, picked up a shopping basket and kicked it along the speckled patterned floor. The shop was packed with young mothers and their grumpy kids, not much younger than Rimi, old ladies pulling tartan patterned trolleys and young couples trying to decide between six chicken drumsticks or six chicken thighs. Rimi drifted down aisle after aisle on the look out. The aisles were stacked high with tins of dog food, cat food and frankfurter sausages. Three different kinds of each. It was by chance that she discovered the eggs tucked away in a corner. Medium, large, brown or white. Which ones to choose? She opened up a carton checking that none were broken. Like baldheads the eggs shone out and Rimi counted them to make sure there were six. Cereal: Shreddies, Rice Krispies, CoCo Pops, Ready Brek, Sugar Puffs or Weetabix. The yellow furry face of the Sugar Puff Monster leapt out at her and Rimi grabbed the packet. Milk: full fat, skimmed, semi skimmed, a pint, a half-pint, a bottle or a carton. Rimi chose a pint in a bottle because that's what the milkman delivered. Bread: brown, white, thick, medium or thinly sliced. Rimi grabbed a small white loaf on the bottom shelf, the only one within reach. Kicking her basket into line Rimi faced the backs of knees. Against a backdrop of voices, crashing trolleys and the ping of the till, she ticked each item off her list slipping the money over the counter; Rimi's head barely reached the top. She slowly packed her bag making sure not to squash the bread. Dragging her bag along the pavement, people didn't seem to notice her diminutive frame. She couldn't reach the front door with the key tied on a string around her neck so she nipped in through the back, unpacked the shopping and left the change on the table. No one asked her to do the shopping. She just did it. Just as every night Rimi set her alarm for school. No one needed to wake her. She never spilt toothpaste on her jumper; she polished her own shoes, tied her own tie and was ready to leave for school by eight. Mina and Amit Bai rarely shouted at her; there was no need. No one worried about Rimi. She was a dream child.

When Bela turned four, Amit Bai and Mina didn't hesitate to send her to Amberleigh to join her big sis. On the first day of term Rimi was ready and dressed, waiting for Bela who was sulking by the wardrobe.

'Why can't I wear my purple dungarees?' Bela whined to Mina.

'Chhuuup, you have to wear a uniform,' Mina waved a tiny shirt at Bela. Seeing the shirt Bela lay on her back in protest and kicked her legs in the air.

'I want to wear my purple dungarees,' she screamed.

A slap on her legs shut her up. Mina continued to wrestle with the petulant four-year old as she tried to run away. After half an hour of sweat, tears and tantrums Bela finally stood in the hallway looking shiny and immaculate in her brand new school uniform, which had cost Mina two weeks wages. Amit Bai couldn't resist taking a photo. Bela pulled a spastic face and then sulked in the corner. She refused to look into the lens until Amit Bai bribed her with a Hubba Bubba. With her mouth full of juicy gum, she smiled an exaggerated smile that verged onto a grimace. Still she looked shiny and dapper in her brand new school uniform and the only thing missing was her front tooth.

Bela didn't cry her eyes out on her first day. She observed all the other kids in their stiff new uniforms, some looked ridiculous in jumpers, too big and shorts too long. Rimi escorted Bela to her classroom and then dumped her there. It was a big, cold room with plastic tables, a black board, red lino floor, white walls and battered wooden chairs. A tall, skinny lady walked in with black hair dotted with dandruff shining like stars. Her name was Miss Flower. She must have been forty-five. Her skin was haggard, features sharp, mouth tight, teeth oversized. Miss Flower scribbled numbers on the board and made everyone recite 2x1=2, 2x2=4. Bela didn't make 2x3=6 because her mind quickly ended up elsewhere in a strange surreal world inhabited by hills made of ice cream and craziness.

On Tuesday morning the infants were taken up a slippery flight of red stairs and told to line up in an orderly line before Miss Flower opened a door and pushed each child in, one by one. Bela walked into a room crammed with hundreds of books. The floor was covered in a honey-coloured carpet, thick and bouncy underfoot and millions of dust particles danced in the shafts of light streaming through the windows. Bela dived into a corner and grabbed a book, spine still intact and pages unblemished. The cover was alive with blond fairies and red spotty mushrooms. She tucked herself into a corner and absorbed the story about a house made of marshmallow inhabited by a tyrannical fat cat called Pumpernickel. She finished that book in fifteen minutes flat. Then she turned her attention to Mr Messy, Mr Strong and Mr Silly. Bela pored over the pictures of curvy landscapes and Mr Silly's brown lace up shoes. After an hour, the other kids started to get restless and disruptive. It was time to return to the blue tables and red tables of the classroom. Bela wanted to disappear into the fluffy carpet with her nice shiny books. She hadn't finished reading Mr Silly. Without thinking twice, Bela slipped the three books up her jumper, folded her arms to conceal the square bulge and filed out. The stairs looked steep and never ending. Bela held onto the banister clutching her tummy with the other. She carefully walked down the stairs, taking her time. She reached the penultimate step, was almost home and dry, until Kevin gave her a push that sent her flying onto the red shiny floor. Miss Flower tried to help her up; Bela didn't move as she felt the books slip out.

Mr Hayden dropped Rimi and Bela off home that same afternoon. Standing in the doorway puffing on his pipe, he stayed an extra five minutes to have a quiet word. He could have been a podgy Sherlock Holmes in his moss felt hat and Burberry scarf. Such a contrast to Amit Bai in his lungi and T-shirt.

Mr Hayden watched Rimi and Bela run past Amit Bai and Mina before turning to the anxious faces of Amit Bai and Mina. The red tufts of Mr Hayden's eyebrows were raised, his voice was low and he talked slowly.

'Rimi, you don't have to worry about. She's a fine student. Really excellent. Bela, well how can I put it, she's developing unhealthy tendencies that need to be kept in check. I don't want to alarm you, but the whole point of a library is to read the books not steal them. Rimi was caught stealing three books. Mr Men books to be exact, Mr Silly, Mr Strong and Mr Square. She said they were her favourite characters but that doesn't mean she can steal the damn things.'

Mina suddenly looked pale and ill.

'Stealing is a of course a very serious offence but on this occasion, on account of her age, she's only four after all, I'll wave the usual punishment for theft.'

'What's that?' whispered Mina.

'Expulsion.'

GUNGI BLUES

Mina and Amit Bai were silent in their shame. Theft at four years old - it was too much to cope with. Bela didn't see taking those Mr Men books as stealing. She was just borrowing them for a while because for the first time in a long time she was enjoying herself and she wanted to prolong the joy for a few more minutes. At least that's how she saw it.

Bela was upstairs, crouched in a ball. The fan heater was on full blast warming up her cold limbs. She wrapped her arms around her head, rocking back and forth ever so slightly. Bela heard footsteps. Heard the door open with a bang and Amit Bai's voice.

'Why did you take those books?' Amit Bai thundered.

Bela didn't respond. She kept her head covered, body crouched. Amit Bai pulled her up by the arms, still entwined around her head.

'You will never ever steal again. Do you understand' Amit Bai shouted thwacking her thighs.

The jagged edge of his ring scratched her thigh and made Bela yelp. Mina watched on as Bela cried begging Daddy to stop. He didn't stop. He couldn't stop. He was trapped in a rage that verged onto slight madness. Bela closed her eyes because Amit Bai's eyes, white and bulging, made her stiff with fear. They finally left. Bela was sniffling. She repositioned the fan heater, locked her arms and rocked, a little harder now. Mina and Amit Bai hoped to dent her consciousness in the right direction with a good beating but beating Bela only left her numb.

The following week Bela flooded the school toilets. She didn't mean to. At first she was simply exploring the inside of the toilet. Then she noticed that if she stopped the ball from rising the water rose creating a lovely waterfall. After Bela didn't return from the toilets, Miss Flower went down to investigate and found her standing in a puddle of water.

'Bela what are you doing?' she shrieked,

'Just seeing how the toilet works,' replied Bela casually.

'Go upstairs right now,' she ordered.

Bela returned to the classroom and sat at her desk. All the other students were scribbling stuff in their notebooks. Bela was quite happy sitting doing nothing. Miss Flower gently tapped Bela on the shoulder and asked

'Is everything OK?'

'Yes miss' smiled Bela.

GUNGI BLUES

'Then do some work!' yelled Miss Flower slamming her hand on the desk.

Bela slowly took out her books. She noticed that her left shoelace was undone and stepped out into the aisle to tie it.

'Bela what are you doing now?' said Miss Flower irritably.

'Doin' my laces Miss.'

'Miss what?'

'Miss Flower.'

Miss Flower looked slightly deranged now and ordered Bela to

'Come out here right now.'

Bela's classmates were deadly quiet. Miss Flower's face was bright red, her black hair ruffled, her lipstick smudged.

'Put out your hand Bela.'

Miss Flower removed a ruler from her desk and smacked Bela's soft pink palm. She flinched and Miss Flower repeated the action.

'Now sit down. I want you to write fifty lines saying 'I must not flood the toilets and disrupt the class. You can write them during break.'

Bela found herself sitting in an empty classroom scribbling her lines, finding it hard to concentrate with the sound of laughing kids in the background.

She didn't flood the toilets ever again. In fact after the ruler she didn't even flush. Bela buckled down to her two times table and she was moved from the blue table for the thickies, who spent most of the day picking their nose and eating snot, to the red table for the supposedly clever kids. Bela still found watching the lollipop lady through the window far more interesting to look at than the back of Miss Flower's head.

It was a week after the toilet incident. Kevin arrived at school fifteen minutes early. Blond with goofy teeth, he was stocky and looked older than his four years. Kevin was jumping about like a frog on acid that morning because today was his birthday. In a Woolworth's bag he carried a family size box of Quality Street. He was going to surprise everyone at lunchtime with his birthday treat and hand out a choc to each kid in class. Like mummy told him to, he left the purple box of chocolates behind the bench in the cloakroom.

Kevin sat at his desk. His knee jumped up and down rapidly with excitement. Bela, who was sitting behind him, raised her hand

GUNGI BLUES

'Please Miss, can I go to the toilet.'

'Off you go, but be quick. I'm timing you.' Miss Flower was busy writing out the four times table on the blackboard.

'Miss.' Repeated Bela.

'What?'

'I think Kevin has got ants in his pants.' The whole class started to laugh and Miss Flower whipped round.

'Kevin stop wiggling!' Kevin couldn't stop. 'Kevin stop that wiggling right now.' Kevin eventually calmed his knees by holding them down but they soon started up again.

The toilets were situated in the cellar next to the cloakroom. It was charcoal black down there, cold and damp. The type of place where serial killers chopped up their victims and hid them under the concrete floor. The drip of a tap echoed in the background and Bela tried to pee quickly. Then she lingered by the coats running her hand against kid's pockets feeling for left over Flying Saucers and Cola Fizzes. She found nothing apart from a leaky biro and bus ticket. Then she saw the Woolworths bag poking out behind the bench. She spotted the purple box of Quality Street shining up at like a precious, wonderful thing. Bela snatched the chocolates out the bag and quite happily claimed the box her own. She examined the list of chocolates. Strawberry Creams, Fudge Crisps, Chocolate Caramel, Mini Milk Chocolate bars and Toffee Twists. Bela licked her lips, she knew she couldn't scoff the lot, nor could she take the chocs home. Instead she devised a plan that would make her the most popular girl in Infant One.

Marching up the stairs, with the purple box of chocs under her arm, she boldly announced;

'It's my birthday and I would like to give everyone a chocolate, two if you're nice.'

Kevin looked bemused as Bela handed out one chocolate each to her classmates. Everyone was beaming at Bela, hoping for an extra choc, and Miss Flower patted her gently on the head for the kind gesture. Bela was the most loved girl in the class until Kevin raced out the classroom. After fifteen minutes, Kevin returned and in between hyperventilating, he said 'Miss, my family box of Quality Street has gone.' Miss Flower called Bela over for a word.

Bela was busily sucking on her long toffee stick to notice. The next thing she knew she was standing in Mr Hayden's office. The worn wooden floors, the wine papered walls, and the fire that raged by his desk made it deceptively warm. Mr Hayden sat in a leather-upholstered chair and Rimi stared at his huge egghead and nasal hair that burned red like the hot coals in the fire. Mr Hayden examined Bela. Her socks lay at her ankles, her shoes scuffed and her jumper, clearly shrunk in the wash, stuck to her body like cling film. She looked quite pathetic. Mr Hayden opened his drawer and pulled out what looked like an old worn slipper. Bela looked at it blankly before Mr Hayden said

'Bela, stand over there and bend over.'

As soon as she bent over, her bottom received a butterfly flurry of sharp, short thwacks. Her tender soft cheeks couldn't quite take the impact. Bela was bawling and her nose was dripping. After the ordeal Mr Hayden calmly put the slipper away and said softly

'It is regrettable that I had to do that but you left me with very little choice. Your parents will be very disappointed in you. I hope that the sting of my slipper will remind you to behave with propriety. As the Head Master of Amberleigh Preparatory School, I have to set an example to the other pupils. It was my duty to punish you. You have done a very mean thing making Kevin cry for two hours on what should have been a very special day. I hope that you have learned your lesson and will try, in the future, to be a good girl like your sister Rimi. Watch and learn from her Bela.'

Bela locked eyes with Mr Hayden and scowled. She returned to a class filled with whispers and stares. She saw Kevin's red and tear stained face.

Bela pulled out her chair, was about to sit down, when Miss Flower said

'Bela you can stand up for the rest of the day.'

Bela didn't mind because her bum was killing her.

'The Slipper' was the worst punishment anyone could get, something you wouldn't wish on your worst enemy, never mind an infant. Mina and Amit Bai sat at the kitchen table, Mina's plait was messy and her face scrubbed clean of make up. The kitchen was in disarray with pots and plates covering the worktop. Washing up, days old, piled up in the sink. A mop in the corner was still swimming in dirty water. Mina didn't seem to care; her attention was fixed on two open photo albums lying on the table.

'What are we going to do?' sighed Mina.

'She needs a good kick' said Amit Bai rubbing his eyes sore from lack of sleep.

Mina pored over photos of Bela when she was a baby. Photos in which she was smiling sweetly, the curls on her head slightly golden, her dimples deep and skin creamy like Ravi's.

'She looks exactly like her father' whispered Mina.

'She looks more like his sister. Probably end up a nutter like her,' Amit Bai said bluntly.

'Don't say that. His sister isn't a nutter, she's just odd.'

'She's a bloody nutter! Ravi told me she was a nutter.'

'No he didn't. Ravi loved his sister, I told you she was a bit strange.'

'She's a nutter and Bela will end up like her if we're not careful' Amit Bai repeated gulping down his tepid tea. 'Look, look at her, pulling those faces.' Said Amit Bai pointing at one photo.

Bela was pulling her trademark spastic face. In another, set against a backdrop of trees, Bela looked lost, oblivious to the camera.

'What I can't understand is that she was the perfect baby.' sighed Mina.

Amit Bai nodded in agreement. 'She just ate, shat and slept. That's my idea of a perfect baby. She was solid, healthy and beautiful,' Amit Bai's eyes trailed away.

'I don't know what to do,' said Mina untangling her hair.

'What she needs is good discipline' snapped Amit Bai.

'Maybe she didn't get enough attention when she was small,' Mina continued to pull at her hair.

'You're right you know. I never picked her up because Ana was always crying that's why Ravi couldn't sleep. Paah, paah, all the time and Bela never complained did she?'

Mina glanced up at the clock. 'You're on the late shift aren't you?'

'Yeah, is there any dhal bhat, I'm so hungry. I only had Sugar Puffs this morning.'

Mina got up and poured a bag of orange lentils into a worn old pan, stained yellow from turmeric. 'We have to do something you know.' Said Mina filling the pan up with water.

' I told you just give her a good kick,' said Amit Bai closing his eyes.

Mina looked at Amit Bai. Strands of silver shone against his black hair, he hadn't shaved and his cheeks sagged. She made him a simple meal of dhal and rice before he went to work. Mina didn't sleep well that night. A storm raged, the rain pelted the windows; the wind battered the walls and her mind raced with too many worries. The next morning, trying hard to hide the emotion in her voice, Mina called the Child Psychiatry Unit at St Mary's hospital.

GUNGI BLUES

Deciding to make it a family outing, Mina made a Saturday appointment. Bela was oblivious to what was really going on and simply thought that she was going to see Dr Roy for some banana-flavoured medicine. For some inane reason Mina and Amit Bai decided to dress Bela up in her best cloths from BHS as if pretty clothes would conceal any traces of latent insanity. She did look sweet in her red fake velvet knickerbockers and lacy frilly shirt. Bela usually had her hair loose in a long thick, knotty mane that moved with a life of its own. Armed with a minuscule comb Mina waded through her hair until it crackled and Bela shrieked. They were just about to leave when Mina asked Bela if she had brushed her teeth. She nodded. Mina didn't believe her and forced her mouth open for a sniff. Her breath was really whiffy. Ordered upstairs Bela rubbed some toothpaste on her gums. She was in a foul mood because she hated obeying anyone, especially, Mina and darted for the front door to avoid further scrutiny but Mina grabbed her by the collar and inspected Bela's face. She noticed that her eyes were still crusty from old sleep. Gobbing a perfect orb of saliva on her finger she laced Bela's eyes with spit and roughly removed the brown muck. Bela tried to squirm out of Mina's firm grip and only after a lot of commotion they finally left. The mood was tense as they walked towards the bus stop to catch the number 44. Amit Bai and Mina were silent in their anticipation that Bela might need serious medication to numb the baby demons breeding in her head. Rimi and Ana didn't really comprehend the gravity of the situation.

As they stood at the bus stop Bela wondered why she was dressed up in velvet knickerbockers while Ana and Rimi looked like a pair of refugees. She wanted to be dressed like a refugee and clawed angrily at her knickerbockers.

The bus chugged along and they all boarded as one big happy family. Little old ladies gave the children gummy smiles and a couple of lonely middle-aged single women became gooey with broodiness. Amit Bai headed for the back seat of the bus but Bela chose to sit on her own in the seat reserved for OAPs and the disabled.

'Bela, come and sit with us,' Amit Bai said sternly.

Bela ignored Amit Bai preferring to scowl at her knees and when they got off Bela walked ten paces behind them.

'Bela come on' Amit Bai yelled.

Bela continued to play deaf as she walked with her head hung down and stared at her patent leather shoes. They were shiny black and perfect. Trying to scuff her shoes she paused to stamp on her feet.

Mina turned round and shouted. 'Bela, what are you doing? Stop that. They're brand new.'

She ignored Mina and continued to stamp on her feet.

They eventually reached the hospital. It loomed tall and fat. A sprawling amalgamation of red brick buildings, far removed from their cosy GP practice with its white washed walls, the rose bushes in the garden and the car park that accommodated only four cars.

'I thought we were going to the doctors,' said Bela.

'We are at the doctors,' replied Amit Bai.

'This isn't the doctors, it's the hospital.'

'It's the same thing,' said Amit Bai.

'No it isn't,' scoffed Bela.

Amit Bai felt a twitch in his hand, a desire to slap Bela's mouth shut, instead he settled for 'Chuuup.'

Inside the hospital the air was heavy and sterile. The walls were shiny and chipped. The doors were old and green. Ana tried to breathe through her mouth to avoid inhalation and closed her eyes to shut out the scary looking sick people but she found she couldn't resist a stare. In front of Ana was an old lady wearing stockings and fluffy slippers. Ana couldn't see her face because her body was bent into a permanent right angle forcing her eyes towards the ground. To Ana’s left was a young mother guiding her skinny boy by the arm; his little finger bound in a bandage bigger than his whole hand. 'Will my finger grow back mummy?' He said. 'Will it mummy?' The young woman anxiously reassured her son with a pat on his head. To Ana's right a middle-aged man in an old tweed suit coughed up a glob of phlegm in his hanky. It was the start of an epic coughing fit that left people turning away in disgust. The place was littered with the ailing old and young and then there was Bela. She looked radiantly healthy, well dressed in her fancy knickerbockers and secure in the company of her whole family.

A black guard in his sixties wearing a well-worn uniform, with white stubble sprouting from his chin, saw them dithering in a corner and offered directions. Inside the lift the walls were carpeted and the ceiling was low. As it squeaked up the floors Bela started to whinge. 'I want to go home. I feel sick.'

'Well, we're going to see a doctor, he'll make you better,' replied Amit Bai

The doors opened at the twelfth floor and they drifted down several pale green corridors before stumbling upon a small waiting room filled with fraught parents and their children. In the middle of the room was a table piled with books and comics, in the corner a bin brimming over with well-used dolls, bricks, and a wooden train. The walls were a shade of bright blue and clashed with the burnt umber carpet. There was even a red beanbag to complement the orange plastic chairs.

GUNGI BLUES

Amit Bai walked up to the receptionist, who was busy scribbling down something in a hardbound notebook. She fashioned a sleek bob with a slither of pink lipstick lining her thin lips. She knew Amit Bai was waiting and kept him waiting several minutes longer before finally looking up 'Can I help you luv?'

'We have an appointment,' said Amit Bai.

'Who's we then?'

'My daughter, Bela.'

'One minute luv, let me check the book. Bela, Bela. Bela. Oh yeah, here we are then. Two o'clock appointment isn't it?' The receptionist looked up at the clock.

'You're fifteen minutes late. Let me just check if that's O.K with the doctor.' After a brief phone call she replaced the receiver and said. 'It's O.K but next time be punctual please. Take a seat luv the doctor will be with you in a minute.'

They all sat down on the slippery plastic chairs. Rimi selected a Beano comic and started to read it quietly. Rimi had managed to find the only decent thing to read so Ana returned to her seat and stared at the other kids. There was one boy with thick curly hair and matching thick eyebrows. He was sucking his thumb and practically squeezing his mother out of her seat. Then there was a blond girl with ringlets who looked like Goldilocks. She was reading a book. It was a thick book with small words and no pictures. Both kids looked perfectly healthy and normal, just like Ana's sister, but perhaps something was lurking in their little minds waiting to pounce out and bite their heads off. Ana turned to examine Bela. She was pulling at her knickerbockers and complained 'Why do I have to wear these? I hate them. I feel stupid.'

'When we get home you can wear something else' whispered Mina.

A bald man with a long moustache, thick bushy eyebrows, round glasses, and corduroy brown pants with a matching jacket and tie called Bela's name. He resembled a tree trunk. Bela turned to look at her parents as Ravi shoved her towards him. She looked puny and pathetic standing next to his long leg.

'I don't want to go,' said Bela.

'Don't be scared? We're right here.'

'Why do I have to go? Why can't they go?'

He was smiling as he put his hand on Bela's shoulder. Rimi and Ana were too busy blowing raspberries at one another to notice Bela staring at them with pleading eyes as the man guided her into his office.

GUNGI BLUES

It was a dimly lit spacious room with a window at the back. There was a soft chair and a table laden with a box of tissues, a sketch book, felt tip pens, crayons and blocks of plasticine - candy pink, breezy blue, toffee brown. In the corner stood an easel with blank paper ready for an attack of paint. Not far from the table was a sink and a towel rack. Against the wall was a family of toys, a zebra, giraffe and cute dolls all arranged as if they knew one another. On a shelf was a modest collection of books propped up against Miss Piggy and Kermit the frog. The room was neatly arranged which made it seem less like a laid back nursery and more like a clinical toyshop.

Bela looked around the room at the soft furry things, the paints, the books and Miss Piggy. She was fixated on the pig and Adam, noticing her fascination, plucked it from the shelf, with his long gangly arm, and gave it to her. Bela took the pig and didn't say thank you. She admired Miss Piggy's purple satin gloves, her upturned snout and long lashes. She wanted to say 'Hi Ya' and do a karate chop but feeling Adam's eyes on her, she stayed quiet.

Adam sat down in his comfy chair and gently said 'Would you like to sit down, Bela?'

Bela did not respond; she was too preoccupied with Miss Piggy's ears.

'Do you like Miss Piggy?' asked Adam in a soft voice.

Bela nodded as she noticed a brand new scuffmark on her left foot.

'Bela, I'm just going to tell you a little bit about myself first. My name is Adam; I talk and listen and try and sort out people's problems. Your mummy and daddy have asked me to have a chat with you about school and home and how you feel about things.'

Bela stayed still and quiet.

'Anything we talk about is just between you and me. OK'

Bela was now investigating Miss Piggy's eyelashes, noticing that they were detachable if she pulled on them very, very hard.

'Bela, I have lots of crayons, pens and paints. Do you like drawing?'

Bela looked over at the table. The brightly coloured pens and big sketchbook looked very inviting and made a change to her lined A4 pad and knackered felt tips. She walked over to the table, sat down, took a fat felt tip and began to draw. The scent of strawberry was a lovely surprise. Perhaps the green felt tip smelt of apple and the yellow of lemon.

GUNGI BLUES

Adam gently pulled up a chair, sat down beside her and asked 'would you like to do some drawings. Maybe of the family?'

Bela stopped drawing and started to sniff the pens instead.

'I know, why don't you just draw a person?'

After a moment of reconsideration, she picked up a black felt tip pen and carefully drew a hexagon with a line sprouting from the top. Underneath the hexagon she added a semi circle. Connecting these shapes with a line she drew a jagged square and dissected it into smaller shapes. Then she made sweeping movements with the black pen drawing swinging arms with boxer glove hands and tiny stick legs. She picked up the red pen and drew another set of arms and intricate shapes with flecks of pink and dots that became a pair of triangular pincers. With the red pen she added a dot on the tip of the line and it stared out like a single eye. With relish Bela coloured the hexagon a deep purple, the semi circle turquoise, the body blue, the hands red. She added other details with rapid strokes and the figure seemed to be jumping, moving, and flailing its arms.

Adam inspected the drawing and said 'very good, Bela but why doesn't it have a nose, mouth or eyes.'

Bela pointed to the red blob on the tip of the stick defensively.

'Oh sorry, is that the eye?' Adam asked.

Bela nodded curtly. Taking a pause, Adam slowly asked 'Is this person sad?'

Bela ignored the question; her concentration was firmly locked on drawing three blocks of black along the bottom of the paper. Refusing to give up, Adam gently coaxed her with the question 'does this person have any friends?'

Finally Bela answered with a firm shake of her head. Growing tired of questions and sweet smelling pens Bela began to wriggle in her chair like a worm stuck in a hole.

'Would you like to do some more drawing. Something else. Anything you like?'

Bela responded to the 'anything you like' and started to scribble a jungle scene of long grass drawing a pink giraffe with ants crawling up its back, a pink duck and a lion in front of an apple tree. There was something floating in the pond next to the lion, a person maybe, it was difficult to tell. And then she used long horizontal strokes for a strip of sky.

Adam only watched and let Bela tear out another piece of paper. She opened a box of pencil crayons and started to draw a pale green scene of curving hills and flecks of grass. It was like a landscape scene in a Mr Men book but without the Mr Men.

He then asked Bela about the drawings; the animals, hills and one-eyed figure but she remained mute. Unfazed by her silence Adam opened a drawer under the table and pulled out a jam jar crammed with scores of multi-coloured pipe cleaners. He pushed them across the table to Bela and she stared at them in wonderment. They looked like skinny furry worms and Bela didn't hesitate to pull one out. Adam pulled one out too and began to bend it into a loop. 'They're fun aren't they?'

Bela took another and another and started to twist and loop the pipe cleaners into a Giacometti stick man.

'Now listen I'd like you to do something. Pretend you are alone on a desert island. If you could choose one person to be with, anyone you like, but just one person, who would that be?'

Bela examined the stick man. It was flimsy and gawky with legs and arms far too long for its short body. Dissatisfied with her creation Bela chucked it. Adam immediately picked up the stick man and sat him carefully on the table. Then he looked Bela in the eye and said

'That must have been scary being thrown onto the floor like that. You know Bela, some people have things that make them feel frightened, I wonder if you have any?'

The question registered something in her head and for the first time she opened her mouth to answer and whispered 'The slipper.'

'What's that?' asked Adam gently.

'It's what you get when you're naughty at school.'

'Tell me about school? Do you like school?'

'No.'

'Why don't you like school?'

'Because I get into trouble.'

'What do you do?'

'I'm naughty and nick books.'

'Why did you nick books?'

'I like books'

'Well I have lots of books you can read for next time. Would you like that?'

Bela nodded but her attention was focused on Kermit the frog. Adam diverted her attention from Kermit by placing the pipe cleaners in front of Bela. She started to pick at them and was soon bending them into strange shapes.

'Lots of people have dreams when they are sleeping at night, I wonder if you do?'

Bela shook her head absentmindedly.

'Often people who don't have dreams like to make up a dream, would you like to do that Bela?'

The thought of dreams triggered something in her head as she twisted and looped the pipe cleaners into abstract wiggles.

'I would like to run away and live with Miss Redfern.'

'Who's Miss Redfern?'

'She's the next-door neighbour.'

'What about mummy and daddy? '

Bela grew quiet before saying

'They'll only be next door. They can visit me'

'Do you like mummy and daddy?'

'No.'

'Why?'

'They make me wear knickerbockers.'

'That must be a pain. I'd like to hear more about that later. Maybe next time you come?'

Adam, seeing that Bela was growing restless with the pipe cleaners, handed her Kermit the frog, which she accepted with a smile. She then proceeded to bash Kermit up with Miss Piggy. Adam observed the scene with interest before gently winding down the session.

Bela emerged from Adam's office clutching twenty pipe cleaners in a vivid array of colours; fuchsia, cyan, deep viridian and ochre. She began to visit Adam on a regular basis and he performed every test in his child psychology textbook. Radiological investigations, computerised axial tomography and psychological tests. Bela didn't mind as long as she always came home with a bunch of pipe cleaners. After three months of intensive tests he concluded that Bela was an extremely intelligent child with a furtive imagination. She was slightly withdrawn with occasional mood swings and that was all. He only suggested that Mina and Amit Bai 'try to be more tolerant and avoid smacking.' He also added that ' in terms of Bela's mental health there is absolutely nothing to worry about. She's a perfectly healthy, bright little girl.'

Amit Bai and Mina were relieved but perhaps they hoped Adam would magic up a fabulous concoction of pills. Pills that would transform Bela into that compliant docile lump of a baby that never gave them any trouble apart from urinating in inconvenient places.

Amit Bai and Mina opted for creative punishment. Smacking was too simple and totally ineffective. If instead they combined a punishment that made Bela think about her actions they might see a significant change in her behaviour. When Bela did something naughty like steal Amit Bai's bus fare or throw half her dinner in the bin Mina shoved Bela's head in the washing machine for ten minutes to make her ponder on her naughtiness. Bela sat with her head in that black hole and watched the speckled walls of the washing machine spin round and round, until the bits of white started to dance around her head. Bela temporarily lost herself in that black hole. She felt like jumping in and splashing around in the blackness until she disappeared. Sometimes she wondered why Mummy put her head in that cold hole in the washing machine but it never made her want to stop being naughty. On the contrary it made her want to annoy Mummy even more.

Under the stairs there was a small pantry where spiders lived in the corners and moths nestled around the light bulb. It was a damp, musty place where Ana's parents stored bags of rice and crates of Fanta. Bela was upstairs squatting in front of the fan heater, wiggling, trying to hold in her wee; too late. A warm stream trickled onto the linoleum floor. Bela went in search of a J-cloth and returned with Mina's ochre silk sari. Bela wiped up the puddle beautifully and left the sari on the floor. When Mina saw her crumpled sari she freaked out. 'Who did this?' She asked knowing it was Bela.

'Did you do this Bela?' Bela stayed quiet and shook her head.

'Don't lie, tell the truth,' Bela slowly nodded and grabbing her by the scruff of the neck Mina pulled Bela downstairs and pushed her into the pantry.

The pantry became a cave filled with huge shadows and monsters. Bela felt something crawling up her leg, but it was just her imagination. She almost instantly started to scream and bawl the place down. The sound of her voice soothed her. If she screamed loud enough perhaps the house would come tumbling down and she could escape to Miss Redfern's. Despite her cries the door remained shut and the walls of the house solid. The only thing that weakened was her red sore throat. Ana heard her screaming and was tempted to let her out but she didn't want to get into trouble. She was too much of a scaredy cat. Bela knew very well that she shouldn't have used Mummy's sari to clean up the wee but now she was glad. Next time she would pour water into Mummy's expensive shoes from Kendals. Mina lay in bed upstairs with her door shut. She was crippled with guilt for hitting and locking her daughter up in the pantry but she would rather let her scream because she couldn't cope with three kids, a job, a new husband and the lingering memory of a dead one. Perhaps Mina wanted to be a caring, sharing, affectionate mother who read her kids Enid Blyton stories and tucked them up at night. She never seemed to have the time. Even though Amit Bai did the washing up, hoovering, shopping and cut onions really finely Mina still had to cook dinner, wash the clothes and do the ironing. She had to sort out the bills, pay the mortgage and hold down a full time job that was miles away. All she really wanted was the very best for her kids and she expected the very best from them.

A couple of days after the pantry incident, Bela stuffed an Asda bag with felt tip pens and a Curly Wurly and slipped though the back door. There was a winding path that led to a field where fat men with hairy legs came out to play football every fortnight. Kids used to roll about in the long grass oblivious to the dog turds hidden beneath the green foliage and when Bela came home one day with an ear full of mud they were banned from the grassy playground and confined to the boring back garden instead. Perhaps this is why Bela chose to roam that field in search of excitement.

There was nothing much apart from wild grass, a weedy path and the odd scruffy sparrow in that field. Bela sat, concealed within a green wall of grass, and drew a picture with her pens. She scribbled with her pink felt tip and munched on her Curly Wurly in a state of bliss. Satisfied with her drawing she packed up her pens and started the long walk down the path. It is strange that no one noticed the little thing bobbing through the grass. The walk was arduous for Bela and her legs began to tire, she needed to go to the toilet and the clouds were welling up in big tufts of grey.

It was not much fun running away but she didn't want to go home for a smack. She sat down on the path and pondered for five seconds before heading back. Her adventure lasted the sum total of fifteen minutes and, although the house was unusually quiet; Bela's parents didn't notice her absence. Set against a dramatic sky the house looked like a strange and scary place. Bela took a detour and rang Miss Redfern's front door bell. Bela's tired, frightened face peeped out behind a messy mass of curls in search of a mint and a friendly face after her failed escape effort. Her knees were mud-stained, the white tips of her socks brown from dirt. Miss Redfern opened the door and when she saw Bela's little face looking up at her she didn't hesitate to usher Bela in. The tired little thing sank into Miss Redfern's silky sofa and Bela began to speak of her adventure. Miss Redfern's house was exactly the same as Bela's in design but inside it was like a spanking new show house. There was not a trace of mess in Miss Redfern's house, not even a stray bit of fluff on the carpet. The smell of Mr Sheen, Murray Mints and Pot Pourri air freshener stuck in the air. Her kitchen was sparkling white like washed snow and her living room was painted in cool olive greens with a delicate pink flower border. Sparsely furnished there was a three-piece suite, an old fashioned TV set which sat in the corner and a small coffee table. On the mantelpiece were two porcelain pelicans and a pair of oriental ducks.

Miss Redfern wasn't prepared for Bangladeshi neighbours and the stench of garlic and fried chilli wafting over her fence. But it was Ravi's death that melted the thick ice block between them. The Christmas after he died Miss Redfern came by the house and gave them a gift of a coffeepot. Amit Bai and Mina didn't drink coffee but they took the gift all the same. She invited them over for sherry and they came round. They ended up sipping out of crystal glasses and nodding when Miss Redfern asked 'top up anyone' even though they thought it tasted vile. Ana and Bela often saw Miss Redfern pruning her roses. She started to smile and chat, grew accustomed to their silly 'Knock Knock, Who's There?' jokes and the screams that pulsated through the thin walls. She knew they were a Gungi family and she didn't judge them. Ana and Bela grew fond of Miss Redfern. They loved to chuck their foam balls over her garden fence just for an excuse to come over for a chat and a sweetie. Other times they would peep over the fence and spy on her. She would jump in fright when she saw their cheeky grins. They were just checking that she wasn't dead. At sixty-five, she was tall, with grey curly hair and long wonky teeth that had yellowed from years of smoking. She weeded and mowed the lawn and went to Asda every Saturday without fail. There was no fear of her dying because Miss Redfern was an old ox and made Amit Bai look like a geriatric.

Miss Redfern listened to Bela, soothing her with Murray mints and somehow the sweetness smudged out the confusion. That's all she wanted, something sweet to suck on and someone to listen. It was growing dark and time slid by as Bela talked and sucked on her fifth mint. The ding-dong of the doorbell made Bela gulp her mint whole. Miss Redfern got up to answer the door. Bela heard voices. She knew it was Amit Bai coming to get her. She thought of hiding but she knew there was no point. Amit Bai appeared in the doorway and within a blink of an eyelid Bela was by his side waving good-bye to Miss Redfern knowing that her adventure was coming to an end.

Amit Bai sent Bela straight up to her room. 'Stay there until I tell you to come out' he ordered.

Bela trudged upstairs to find Rimi on the landing blowing raspberries on Ana's stomach. She stepped over them, turned on the fan heater and indulged in her favourite past time. Warming her bum. Rimi was tickling Ana without mercy and she started to scream with laughter. Clasping her ears, Bela tried to block out the sounds. Rimi continued to tickle Ana and she continued to shriek. Secretly, Bela wanted to be tickled and tortured. Why didn't they play with her? Why was she sitting alone in a cold bedroom on the hard lino floor getting a burnt bum? Why was she born in the middle? For what? The middle child was a misfit. The problem child. The one who ran away and nicked Mr Men books. Tears stung like the juice of a lime nestling in the slit of a fine cut and she started to bite her nails until there was nothing left to bite on. No one can be sure when her nail biting actually started. People assume that nail biting is a product of too much nervous tension. Something that people with furrowed brows do at bus stops when they're running ten minutes late. Or an absent minded habit that comes from boredom. Whatever Bela's reason she started to bite her nails with the hunger of a child who has missed their breakfast. Nibbled at untidy loose skin, tore it away in thin strips until her fingers bled. Bela wrapped her tongue around those salty red beads. Sinking in the saltiness. Dancing on the high of the pain. When she'd finished feasting, her fingers were left dangling like lacerated bodies by her sides.

The day Ana started Amberleigh fulfilled her parents' dream of sending all their kids to private school. To capture the moment, they stood outside the house, dressed in shiny red uniforms and grinned into the camera for Amit Bai. For the next seven years Ana's parents could relax and let Mr Hayden take care of the rest. Mina didn't have to worry about dropping them off at school either because Aunty Pat kindly gave them a lift. Both her children, David and Rebecca, went to Amberleigh and didn't live far. Aunty Pat said it would be a pleasure to take the three of them to school as long as Mina paid her a few quid.

Aunty Pat was a beautiful woman with jet-black curly hair and sexy legs. She wore low cut transparent shirts that flashed her wrinkled, freckled cleavage to the world. Aunty Pat's husband left her for a younger woman when Rebecca was three. She was devastated but her eyes never lost their sparkle. It was odd that such a slender and elegant frame could produce two fatties. David was soft and round and Rebecca, at four years old, resembled a Weeble. Every morning the three of them would squeeze into the back of the car. Rebecca took up at least two seats leaving the others squashed together in an uncomfortable tangle. And if Ana's leg dared touch hers Rebecca would pinch her hard with her piggy fingers.

It was Monday morning and Rebecca was flicking Ana's leg with a ruler. Ana politely pushed her hand away. The flicking continued and Ana's leg began to blush. Rimi gave Ana a big sister look of reassurance and then ignored the situation. Bela seemed to enjoy Ana's pain. Aunty Pat was singing along to some obscure Elvis Presley track and David was snoring. A quiet rage simmered in Ana's belly. The next thing she knew Ana's fist landed in Rebecca's ocean of fat and dissolved in her tyres. Rebecca screamed. Aunty Pat slammed on the brakes. Everyone jerked forward and the car behind crashed into Aunty Pat's back bumper. That same day Aunty Pat came over to the house and said that 'on second thoughts, there isn't enough room in the car for six. I don't think I can pick up the kids anymore'.

Aunty Pat left before Mina and Amit Bai could ask any questions so they queried the children afterwards. Ana was hoping for solidarity. Rimi acted dumb, Ana remained silent and Bela said 'She...' said Bela pointing at Ana 'she punched Rebecca in the tummy; that's why Aunty Pat's car got wrecked.'

Amit Bai glared at Ana 'you idiot. Now how will you get to school, hey?' Ana tensed up and prepared for a slap across the cheek. Fortunately, Amit Bai calmed down, Ana escaped the slap and Bela looked peeved.

With no more Aunty Pat, Amit Bai put an ad in the Manchester Evening News for a child minder.

'These kids need proper discipline. Some one to pick them up, feed them and sort them out' he said.

They couldn't understand why Mina and Amit Bai were going to pay for some strange person to come into the house and order them like dogs. They liked their simple life. Got home, got changed, watched telly wrecked the house and fought like monkeys. Turned the bedroom upside down. Played dead with their tongues hanging out. Jumped up and down on the sofa to the beat of Pakeezah. Skied down pillow dunes. Watched the TV screen shrink to a white dot and disappear with a blink. This was their life.

A pair of red haired freckled twins first responded to the ad. They arrived on the doorstep chewing gum, wearing tight jeans, red lipstick and strode into the house without wiping their trainers. They told Mina and Amit Bai that they had "loads of experience", "loved kids" and that their hourly rate was "fifty pee". Amit Bai never called them back. A week later Mrs Bond arrived, wearing thick blue glasses with her hair neatly set in silver white curls. She was a robust sixty-five year old with stocky legs, strong freckled arms, twitching fingers and skin the colour of dirty dishwater. Mina and Amit Bai called the children downstairs to introduce them to their new child minder. Mrs Bond smiled sweetly at them as she sipped tea and nibbled on a biscuit.

The following Wednesday Mrs Bond picked them up from school. Three brown kiddies walking with an old white lady. It looked strange and felt weird. They arrived home and Mrs Bond said ‘hurry up and get changed. Tea’ll be ready in a minute.’

They peeled off their uniform as the smell of over boiled peas and hot chip fat wafted upstairs. After twenty minutes they heard the shrill cry of Mrs Bond, ‘tea’s ready.’

GUNGI BLUES

Bela had just removed her tie and was in no particular hurry. Rimi and Ana, slightly fearful of the woman, flung on some clothes and ran downstairs. They heard the music of Jackanory in the background. They would have much rather watched telly, instead they walked into the kitchen. Waiting for them were stodgy chips, peas and fish fingers. No rice, no dhal, no roast chicken, no spicy salad, no chillies to chew on, no food to make their noses run with snot and eyes water buckets.

'Well don't just stare at it, sit down and eat,' barked Mrs Bond.

There was still no sign of Bela and Mrs Bond began to mutter 'her tea's getting stone cold.'

She called Bela again; there was no reply. Losing patience, Mrs Bond marched upstairs and found Bela rocking in front of the fan heater, still wearing her uniform. 'What on earth are you doing?'

'I'm cold' mumbled Bela.

'Get up you daft thing, turn off that heater and come downstairs.' Bela pulled a face, got up slowly and followed Mrs Bond out the room.

The three of them now sat at the kitchen table picking at their food.

Rimi whispered 'There's a hair in my baked beans.'

Bela complained 'My fish fingers taste of old J Cloths.'

And Mrs Bond interjected with 'No talking at the table and no one leaves until you finish every last pea on your plate'.

Ana attempted to cut a fish finger. It was rock hard forcing her elbows up and down like a flapping chicken. Mrs Bond snapped 'Keep your elbows in and hold your knife and fork properly. It's not a shovel you know.'

Ana wanted to eat her peas with her hands, burp and tell silly jokes.

'But Mrs Bond...' Ana said with a mouth full of fish finger.

'Don't talk with your mouth full and keep your elbows in,' said Mrs Bond holding her elbows down as she tried to cut her chips.

'That's better,' Mrs Bond said triumphantly and returned to her soaking dishes.

Once Mrs Bond's back was turned Bela stuffed chips down her jumper in protest. Rimi spat out half chewed food in her kitchen towel, folded it neatly into a dainty parcel and slipped it in her pocket. Somehow they all managed to clear their plates without consuming much food. The ordeal was not over. There was still desert. Pink Angel Delight. Sickly sweet, the texture of snot.

With heavy stomachs, they finally got up to leave.

'Erm excuse me, haven't you forgotten something?' said Mrs Bond.

They looked at one another and Rimi said 'I don't think so.'

Mrs Bond sighed 'hasn't your mother taught you to say 'Please may I leave the table?'

They shook their heads. Mrs Bond stopped drying her bunch of forks and sighed. 'Never, ever leave the table without being excused. It's bad manners. Got it. So what do you say then?' Said Mrs Bond clapping her hands in expectation.

'Please may I leave the table Mrs Bond. Thank you for the lovely tea. It was very nice' said Rimi sweetly without hesitation.

Ana tried to emulate her big sister and Bela grunted inaudibly. It felt odd asking to leave the table in their own home. Felt alien. Felt outrageous.

Ana opened her eyes and watched Mina who was deep in sleep. The frown in her brow softened. Her left foot trailed the floor as she snored slightly and Ana lifted it up and put it back under the duvet. Ana tip toed out and saw Amit Bai was snoozing in the spare room with the paper nestling on his belly rising and falling to the rhythm of his breathing. The kitchen was a mess with pots and pans covering the work surface. The floor covered in onion peel and chilli ends. She walked through the green hallway, past the purple bathroom to the small room where she sat on the bed to reflect. What would life have been like without the three of them? Quiet and financially more rewarding. Ana tried to rationalise her mother's grief and how it impacted on them as they grew up. Her melancholy seeped into their blood and they lived and breathed sadness. Ana couldn't blame either of them though. 'They did their best' Ana concluded. Hiring a woman like Mrs Bond wasn't cheap. It was a financial strain. They thought that Mrs Bond would instil them with discipline and etiquette. Her presence only made home more like a prison, a place full of ridiculous rules, a place where they could no longer run wild and scream. Mrs Bond silenced the child in them and smothered their spirit.

John Craven's Newsround was ending and Blue Peter was about to start. They sat on the sofa with their feet on the table, glued to the box. Mrs Bond walked in and said 'Why don't you do some drawing instead of watching TV? Go on, go upstairs and get your felt tips.'

They didn't have much choice. Mrs Bond made them sit with their backs to the television and draw beach side happy family scenes. This whole exercise was not about artistic edification. It was her way of watching Countdown in peace while they ended up watching the gaping hole between her legs. The flesh of her thighs was pink and flabby. The point at which her thighs met dark and scary. So scary that Ana looked away and picked up a felt tip for solace. Rimi was drawing a smiling child eating ice cream in the sun. Bela was busy completing the horns of her monster. He was wrestling with a man wearing a string vest and underpants. Standing by the palm tree was a woman, beating a baby, with her handbag. After Countdown Mrs Bond inspected the work. She smiled and said ‘clever girls’ to Rimi and Ana. Mrs Bond examined Bela’s effort. She frowned and said nothing. Bela wanted a response, a word, a comment, but not silence.

It was a warm and balmy September afternoon. Sitting on the bus home they tore off their thick woolly jumpers and picked at their socks. After another diabolical tea Mrs Bond said ‘go and play in the garden. The fresh air will do you good.’

Bela asked softly ‘Mrs Bond, please may I go upstairs and get my books?’

‘Of course sweetie pie,’ replied Mrs Bond somewhat surprised that Bela said ‘please.’

Bela returned with three Mr Pinkwhistle books, a teddy bear, duvet, two jigsaws and an old sari. They draped themselves in silk. Took turns playing mummies. Made Bela lay down on the sari and wrapped her up tight. Her body squirmed and they laughed until they heard her muffled cries and were forced to unwrap her. Pale and dripping with sweat Bela gasped

'I couldn't breath. You nearly killed me' and sulked off to the garage.

The garage was bigger than the sitting room. A hoard of junk, a broken old lawn mower, plywood, battered boxes and rusting tools created jagged silhouettes, cracks of dark and thick piles of dust. Bela poked around in one box and discovered a pile of mags. On the front cover was a blond lady with her white breasts hanging out. Wearing tiny turquoise bikini bottoms, she stood next to a tanned man wearing a black pouch. Bela turned the pages one by one and saw blonde ladies, pale boobs, wobbly bums and plastic grins. Sneaking upstairs she locked herself in the toilet to pore over the funny hair does and fake tans without risk of discovery. Each picture left Bela warm and tingly inside.

Mrs Bond was busy mopping the kitchen floor. A lovely blue, trapped behind years of dirt, shone through and made her smile with pride. Once finished she fixed herself a cup of tea and sat down to watch the Countdown final. During the commercial break, Mrs Bond fancied a digestive to dip in her tea. She was greeted by a pitter-patter of dirty footprints on her nice clean floor. Enraged,

GUNGI BLUES

Mrs Bond ran into the garden, where Rimi and Ana were inanely pulling out grass, and demanded to know who messed up her 'nice clean floor.' They shook their heads indifferently and continued to tear at the grass. Mrs Bond ran inside and called for Bela who acted deaf as she sat on the toilet, glued to a picture of a man with his leg cocked in the air. After two minutes of shouting Mrs Bond ran upstairs. Hearing the rustle of a turning page Mrs Bond pounded on the toilet door. Bela didn't budge.

'Open this door this instant' Mrs Bond shrieked.

Bela flipped over the next page. After standing outside the toilet door for ten minutes, yelling, banging and pounding, Mrs Bond accepted defeat and went downstairs to make another cup of Tetley's to calm her nerves. An hour elapsed. Bela was still in the toilet. Mrs Bond's knees began to quiver as her bladder swelled with swishing tea. Bursting, she ran upstairs and demanded entry. Bela hid the magazine behind the loo; let Mrs Bond sweat for another five before finally opening the door. The desperate woman pushed Bela out the way, pulled down her knickers and let it all out with a sigh. Mrs Bond couldn't wait to scold Bela but Bela was on another trip. Words did not seem to penetrate. She'd heard it all before. 'You're a bad, bad girl,' 'wicked' and 'malicious.' Bela was past caring. She was born to defy and laugh in the face of silly rules and pathetic orders. Frustrated, Mrs Bond started to shake Bela until her soft brown cheeks quivered. Bela remained mute, her expression empty. In the end Mrs Bond gave up and discarded Bela to one side like a tube of empty toilet roll.

Ana and her sisters soon learnt that if they obeyed Mrs Bond like good little girls, life would be sweet like Angel Delight. Mrs Bond was unable to pick them up from school on Wednesday because she was having a purple rinse at the hairdresser's the same day. She couldn't possibly cancel because it was Howard's wedding the following Sunday. Howard was Mrs Bond's only son and she loved to talk about his 'fancy job', 'his brand new Escort' and how she was 'thankful to the lord for such a peach of a son'. Mrs Bond warned them on the Tuesday during Tea that 'under no circumstances do you get off at the main road, it's too dangerous. Get off at the stop before and cross at the traffic lights. Don't groan Bela. It's only a five minute walk.' It was more like twenty actually. 'I'll be waiting for you at home after I've had my hair rinsed.'

They sat on the bus that chilly Wednesday afternoon. The streets were lined with ice and dirty sheets of sleet. They shivered in their duffel coats and their knees were bleached white with cold. Their stop came but none of them moved an inch and they casually got off at the forbidden main road, where cars zoomed too close to the kerb and loomed like massive metal monsters. Rimi looked unfazed, held her sisters' hands tight, told them to stand in line, looked right, then left and said 'after three, run.'

Half-screaming they made a mad dash to the other side and once safely across they cheered and laughed, jumped and slapped each others backs, Amit Bai style. To play it extra safe, they crawled by the side of the wall to conceal the direction they were coming from. Their knees stuck to the icy pavement and hands stung with pain. They were almost home until Ana saw a pair of familiar blue leather shoes and looked up to see Mrs Bond looming over her. In the winter light Mrs Bond's hair shone cerulean blue and hundreds of tight curls crawled over her head. She looked like an alien on the verge of zapping Ana with its curly antennae.

'I told you to get off at the traffic lights. You can turn right round and walk back to the bus stop.' They all stared at her thinking she was joking. Mrs Bond's fat wet lips remained sour.'Go on, off you go. That'll teach you. And listen I'm timing you so don't pull any stunts.'

The three of them didn't argue with her. Miserable, wet and freezing they walked back. Twenty minutes later, they saw the sweet shop on the corner. It looked warm and inviting. Rimi peered into her tiny purse and produced ten pee. Ten pee could buy a bus ride home, a Milky Way and ten sweeties, even more if you bought half penny chews. They filed into the shop. A round smiling lady stood behind the counter and a Chihuahua, dressed in tartan with its hair tied up in ribbons, snoozed in its basket.

Bela caressed the Mars Bars, Marathons, Crunchies and Yorkies with a finger. Rimi ignored them; they were beyond her price range. Sitting behind a well-polished glass window scores of sweeties stared up from their plastic homes. Teddy bears, banana chews, black jacks, drum sticks, cherry lace, bon bons and half penny sweeties. Bela drooled and Ana watched greedily as Rimi contemplated her selection. After ten minutes of deliberation Rimi made her final choice.

'One Flying Saucer, one Banana Chew, one Cola Fizz, one Cola Bottle, two Mint Mojos, one pink Bon Bon, yes that's right, one Black Jack and two Teddy Bears, one red and one green, please.'

It was an inspired choice. They left the shop and Rimi carefully dropped the sweeties into their frozen palms. The little sweeties stared up crying out to be gobbled up. The sherbet in the Flying Saucer zapped the cold in her ears and the pink chew of the drumstick stuck to her teeth, Bela consumed hers in less, while Rimi made her sweets last all the way home.

Mrs Bond pounced on Amit Bai as he walked through the door. She couldn't wait to tell him about the naughty defiance. On and on she droned and Amit Bai nodded wearily. After a punishing fourteen-hour night shift Amit Bai was puffy eyed and sleepy. He wasn't listening to Mrs Bond because he wasn't interested in how naughty they were; all he wanted to do was sleep. Mrs Bond left after another cup of tea and half a packet of Rich Tea biscuits. Ana and Bela expected stern looks and reprimands from Amit Bai, but all they got was 'go up-stairs, do your homework and no funny business. I'm going to bed.'

Now that Mrs Bond had gone Ana and her sisters flushed social etiquette down the toilet and the irrepressible animal in them reared its ugly head. Despite the warning, the urge to play noisy, violent games was too great. Bela and Ana started to chase each other round the onyx table to the tunes of Runa La La. Faster and faster until painful stitches left them curled up on the floor. An old broom became the horse and they cried 'Get off your horse and drink your milk' in dubious John Wayne accents as they rode up and down getting splinters in their skin. They sprayed the linoleum bedroom floor with shoe polish, transforming their room into a rink and skated in their socks. They even made up a song

Johnny Briggs
Superstar
Looks Like a woman coz he wears a wig
The wig's too big
So he wears a bra
That's why they call him a dirty pig

Ana and Bela sang Johnny Briggs in silly voices and laughed their heads off until their bellies ached and couldn't take any more. They were making a racket and Ana suggested 'Bela we'd better keep it down.'

All smiles and white teeth only seconds before Bela's face suddenly turned cold 'Why don't you keep it down yourself.'

'I am' Ana said in a loud whisper.

'No you're not' shouted Bela.

'Shhh, he'll wake up and then we'll get it.'

'Why don't you shut up then?' said Bela with her face inches from Ana's.

'I am' Ana said backing away.

'No, you keep on going on,' said Bela edging forward.

'Bela just shut it.' Ana said pushing her back.

'Don't tell me to shut it you stupid cow and don't push me,' said Bela poking Ana in the shoulder.

'Get off me you, you fat pig.'

'You know why I can't stand you? I can't stand you because you always ruin it.' Bela glared at Ana. Her face was creased up in lines, like an old woman.

Ana decided to ignore her. Play with her Lego instead. And she started to adjust her plastic flowers and trees.

'Oi.' Bela said grabbing Ana by the shoulder 'Don't ignore me when I'm talking to you?'

Ana tried to concentrate on the red and yellow flowers.

'Stop playing with your stupid Lego' said Bela poking Ana again.

That poke triggered something inside. Ana turned around and gripped Bela's lovely soft arms. Her nails dug deep into her creamy flesh. Bela's fingers pulled at Ana's hair. Ana dug deeper until she saw shavings of curled skin, swollen bumps and speckles of blood dotting Bela's arms. Bela shook herself free, picked up a Lego house and threw it to the ground. It was the one with lights, fridge, cooker and table. It was Ana's favourite Lego house and now it lay in fragments. Ana reached for Bela's face. Her eyes, nose and mouth twisted up in her hand. Bela started to scream. The smell of interrupted sleep wafted into the bedroom and Amit Bai appeared. His hair stood on end, the whites of his eyeballs were completely blood red and his hairy belly quivered under his shrunken T-shirt. As Amit Bai advanced towards them they ran into the bedroom. Bela climbed onto her bed and tried to hide under the duvet. Tears were already streaming down her cheeks and Amit Bai hadn't even laid a finger on her. Bela started to beg 'Please don't hit me. Please daddy.'

Ana curled into a ball and waited for a dose of pain. She heard his footsteps, his heavy breath and the pause before the sharp thwack to the head. Bela got a couple of slaps. Slaps that made her scream exaggerated screams. Then Amit Bai said 'anymore fighting and I'll give you another kick.' And left.

Bela and Ana were silent for about two minutes. 'This is all your fault.' Muttered Bela. 'Have you seen what you've done to my arms you animal?'

'Let's not start again.' Ana pleaded trying to hold back her tears as she attempted to reconstruct the foundations of her Lego house.

Predictably within minutes of the slap Bela and Ana were squabbling again. Things that Ana did months ago suddenly became new points of contention. Books of hers that Ana had read without her permission. Felt tip pens that Ana had abused. Sweets that Ana had stolen from her blazer pocket. The fight was escalating and Ana was defending her innocence even though she knew she was guilty. Amit Bai re-appeared. She automatically curled herself into a small ball once more. Bela squealed like a pig and pleaded with Amit Bai not to hit her. Somehow Amit Bai's foot found Ana's head and she felt a kick, mightier than a footballer's. Ana's head jutted forward and she tried to rub away the pain with her hands. She heard the thump of Amit Bai's fist across Bela's back. Her cries made Ana's head hurt. She did not make a sound. After five minutes Amit Bai left them to stroke their sore spots better.

Fighting with Bela was a habitual feature of Ana's life from the age of six onwards. She didn't want to fight with her, Ana wanted to be her twin, dress like her, look like her and be like her. Ana admired the way Bela never got splash marks on the backs of her white socks, her beautiful thick curly hair, her dimples, her fat lips, her hazel eyes and her use of words like 'docile' at the age of seven. She wanted to play with her at Amberleigh even though she pretended they weren't related. She liked their games. Reading the dictionary. Laughing about silly words like 'ennui'. Pressing their tummies on the cold surface of the TV screen for titillation. Drinking Bovril in deck chairs outside the house and waving at the passersby. If Bela was in the mood to play it was sublime but often playtime with Bela turned into a twisted power game.

It was a Sunday afternoon. There was nothing to do. Ana fancied a game of chase, anything really. She went in search of Bela and found her sprawled out on the bed

'Bela will you play with me?' Bela acted deaf.

'Bela, will you play with me?' Ana repeated. Bela looked up and after a ridiculous pause said coolly

'If you make me a sandwich, yeah I'll play with you.'

Ana went downstairs and made her a sandwich with tomato, lettuce, turkey and whole grain mustard. She prepared it with care and a little love. Then Ana hand delivered the sandwich with a glass of milk and watched Bela munch it down without an utterance of thanks.

'So will you play with me now?' Ana asked getting slightly impatient. Bela shook the crumbs from her red skirt before saying 'Only if you clean my shoes first.'

Ana was getting desperate now but the situation was a little like waiting for the bus. You know that if you give up and start walking the bus will come and you'll be annoyed because you missed it by half a second. Instead you endure the bite of the cold for another half-hour in the hope that the bus will soon chug along and take you to where you want to be. So without a word Ana collected her shoes and buffed away the scuffs.

'I've cleaned your shoes, now will you play.' Ana said holding up the gleaming black things. Bela didn't even bother to look up because she was too engrossed in Charlie and Chocolate Factory.

'Tidy up my books first, then we'll see.'

GUNGI BLUES

Ana didn't mind tidying her books because she liked to arrange things in nice orderly piles. Once she finished Ana came bouncing back to her sister who was now downstairs watching the Price Is Right with Bruce Forsythe.

'Can we play now?'

'I want to watch telly. We'll play tomorrow, promise.'

Rather than kick her head in Ana utilised the rest of an otherwise wasted day and skipped one thousand skips in the yard.

Ana didn't blame Bela for fobbing her off with lame excuses. Why should she play with her? Ana was the one who got the top bunk. She took up most of the floor with the castles; spaceships, trucks, cars, post office and petrol pump that made up her sprawling Lego town. She cried if Amit Bai didn't buy her the latest train set even though it was sixty-five pounds. Bela never asked for anything much. She still slept with the teddy given to her at aged three. Teddy only had one eye, his creamy fur was flat and bald in patches, but Bela dressed Teddy in a red jumper, clung to him at night, and never asked for a new one. If Teddy belonged to Ana she would have binned him years ago. They were at odds. Turned on by different things. The only common denominator was the violence subjected to them on a weekly basis. After a fight, Bela would sulk, refusing to wipe her glistening snot trails and tear stained cheeks. Ana would let her cool down for a few hours before pulling a silly face that made Bela smile, then she'd say 'sorry' in a childish voice. Sorry was the magic word that made them friends once more. Reconciliation was temporary, the peace between them precarious, but within those brief moments they were close.

After a while, Ana became used to the kicks and immune to the pain. Hitting in public was far worse than hitting at home. The fundamental difference between private and public beating was that only you and the beater knew about it.

It was Saturday afternoon. The whole family had just got off the number 43 bus at Piccadilly station. Town was teeming with people, there was a long queue at the chippy and the smell of vinegar and hot potato was making Ana hungry. Amit Bai and Mina pushed their way towards the Arndale. The Arndale centre had become a place for teenagers to show off their latest trainers, shell suits and greasy perms. It was a place to suck fags and cop off. Ana was holding Amit Bai's hand as they entered Marks and Spencers. Crowded, noisy and sweaty, Ana already wanted to go home. She dawdled by some blue dresses with flower shaped buttons. If Ana pulled hard enough the button would come off and she could slip it in her pocket. No one would know. The rest of the family were walking towards the escalators. 'Come on.' Shouted Mina in a voice she dare not disobey. She couldn't help glancing back at those buttons.

GUNGI BLUES

'Can we come back later?' Ana asked pulling at Mina's plait. 'Can I?' Ana asked pulling again.

Ana should have realised that Mina was hassled. It could have been anything, something Ana said. Something she did, like pulling her plait a little too hard. Sure enough she saw Mina's hand rise. Ana ducked and hoped that people might think Mina was swatting a nasty fly but she clipped the back of Ana head. She went flying forward and, losing her balance she fell into the immaculate line of navy dresses. The M&S lady looked peeved. Ana felt like she had committed a terrible offence and everyone else thought Ana was a small piece of scum lying in a sewer. Ana wanted to hide amongst those dresses and mutate into a button. Ana could see the pity in people's eyes. She tried to focus on the tip of her shoe, could feel her self-esteem shrink to the size of a rice grain and for the rest of the day Ana felt like shit.

It was the evening of the Christmas school play. Ana was acting the obscure part of the badger in Goldilocks and the three bears. Even though Ana knew that the part was an invented one, she didn't care. Ana was proud to wear her badger's mask and prance about the stage like a little plonker. The school hall was packed with parents including Ana's. It was ten minutes before curtain rise and Ana was still dressed in her school uniform. She started to strip off frantically until Ana was standing in her vest, knickers and lace up shoes. She struggled to put on her leotard with its annoying strappy bits and the mask was fiddly with detachable ears. Once Miss Flower Sellotaped the mask to her head, Ana was a proper badger and stood in line between frog and fox. Miss Flower gave Ana the crucial OK signal and she bumbled on stage. She performed a cute thirty-second dance with the rest of the animals and then crouched by a cardboard bush for the rest of the evening. Ana searched for her parents in the dark, eager for a glimpse of their proud faces but she only saw shadows and murky figures. By the end of the play Ana had cramp and sore knees but she couldn't resist mingling with the audience to show off her badger mask and bobbly tale. When Ana got back to the changing room she found everyone dressed and ready to leave with their parents'. Ana lazily flung her uniform over her leotard and tried to slip her feet into her shoes. The sound of 'hurry up, we'll miss the bus home' made Ana freeze. Amit Bai was standing behind her. Parents, teachers and pupils were staring, Amit Bai was fast losing patience and Ana was battling with laces and shoes. She saw the rising hand of Amit Bai. Hoped he might reconsider. Too late. A hard swipe graced the back of her head. Everyone saw it.

Ana was glad when Amit Bai pushed her out of the packed changing room because she wanted to escape. On the way home Amit Bai suggested that they stop off for some 'chips and fish'. Smiling and munching on cod Amit Bai had clearly forgotten the slap. To him it was just a small tap on the head. No big deal. No long-term brain damage or anything.

Nothing compared to the beatings he received from his mother in Barisal.

Ana tried to give Amit Bai the silent treatment but he wouldn't stop pestering her with 'you were very good you know, but why was your part so little.' Ana didn't answer.

Amit Bai persisted until Ana responded. There was no sorry for the slap and there was no point demanding an apology. These public outbursts of violence were a part of life. Something the children brought on themselves. Something they couldn't question because their parents didn't have any answers it was just the way it was.

Secondary School

Rimi was eleven, Bela eight and Ana was seven years old. It was time for Rimi to leave the safe cosy haven of Amberleigh and enter the scary secondary phase of education. For two solid weeks Rimi took fourteen entrance exams and received offers from every single one: Stretford Grammar, Altrincham Grammar, Withington High - there were too many to choose from but there was no contest. With a reputation as an efficient super brain-manufacturing machine Rimi was going to Manchester High. If it meant Rimi getting into Oxford the high fees didn't matter. Amit Bai decided to put Bela forward for the entrance exam at Manchester High too. Maybe then she'd stop 'sitting on her arse' and do some work. Bela passed the exam without trying and in the space of a fortnight Bela was taken out of Amberleigh and scheduled to start her first term at Manchester High with Rimi.

Manchester High didn't have a cute dinner lady serving soggy jam sponge with custard. Six buildings made up the school, one of which housed a swimming pool. The entrance was grand with a sweeping staircase and the stench of elitism stained the air. Amit Bai and Mina forked out a small fortune on new uniforms, PE kits and neatly sewn nametags. The blazer was liquorice black with a puke yellow border, the skirt was black, the shirt custard yellow topped off with a black hat. It was a sad day for Ana on 9th September because as Ana walked with her sisters down the road Ana turned left towards the bus stop and they turned right instead. Ana watched Bela pause mid way. She took off her shoe and itched her foot, then she fumbled in her knickers and produced a stray long hair that had nestled in her bum crack. She looked back, smiled, and waved the hair at Ana. It was a poignant moment that not many would understand.

From day one Bela was lost in that maze of a school. Everyone had his or her established network of friends and Bela was the new kid. Awkward, shy and withdrawn she was the perfect target for bullies. No one made her feel welcome or warm inside. At first she tried to make polite conversation with the others but they ignored her as soon as she opened her mouth. There was no explanation for the dirty looks or the silent treatment. Bela tried to rationalise the hostility thinking she had bad breath. Either that or the entire school was full of snobs. Bela pined for Amberleigh, the small playground and her old classroom with the squeaky floorboards. At Amberleigh she used to go to her special corner where she fiddled with bits of twig and mud. Now she stood alone, in a vast concrete expanse, looking down at her scuffed shoes. There were hundreds of Sherber Dab kids scurrying in every direction like ants on speed. Without any warning Bela needed to go to the toilet, although she had only just been. Before she knew it she felt an ocean break through her clenched lips. A hot loud trickle slid down her leg staining her white ankle socks and she stood with her shoes submerged in a pretty puddle not knowing what to do. One moment she was an insignificant dot now all eyes were on her and she faced smirking faces and embarrassed whispers. Bela sought comfort within the smelly confines of the school toilets. Sobbing on the bog, two little bitches peeped over and started cursing her

'Shit for brains, short arse, arse wipe, smelly knickers, soggy knickers.'

Bela wanted to shout back and scour their blue eyes out with two rusty kebab skewers. She wanted them to hurt inside but her mouth refused to open.

To cope with the loneliness and the nasty nameless faces Bela buried herself in books. The library at Manchester High was in the super league and Bela felt she'd landed in heaven when she first saw the impressive room with wooden trimmings, high ceilings and potted plants. She started to spend hours there losing herself in fantasy worlds of castles, silly kings and petulant princesses.

It was a cold, windy afternoon and Bela was waiting for Rimi in the library. Beside her were three juicy books that she liked the look of with their hard back shiny covers and sophisticated illustrations but the book that captured her interest was an anthology of Larkin's poetry. It somehow ended up in the wrong book section and landed in Bela's lap. Most of the poems she didn't really understand. Too packed with irony and hidden meanings however, there was one poem that stuck out like a flashing red beacon with its opening line

'They fuck you up your mum and dad, they may not mean to but they do. They fill you with the faults they had and add some extra, just for you.'

These words were like a revelation. It wasn't her fault that people picked on her and made her life hell. Her parents were the culpable ones. They were the ones who yelled at her for any small reason and gave her a wallop every day for nothing. Her misery stemmed from the misery they inflicted on her. She was unpopular because her parents made her feel rotten, that's why kids said she stank of mouldy veg. It was easy to blame them and it felt good to blame them for everything that was going wrong in her life. Bela wanted more revelations but the library was closing. She already had six books out and she wasn't allowed anymore. No one would notice if she just slipped the book in her satchel and returned it the following week. She promised herself that she would.

The next day Bela was called out of class to the Head's office. Mrs Rosenthal was sitting at her oak desk caressing a silver Parker between thumb and forefinger. Her office was sparse with a few select placards on the wall and a small bookcase on the side, jam-packed with leather bound books that had never been read. Mrs Rosenthal spoke to Bela in a voice that tried to hide the Oldham tinge in her accent.

'Yesterday, you were in the library weren't you?'

Bela nodded.

'Well apparently Bela a book has been reported missing: a book of Larkin's poetry. Do you know anything about it?' said Mrs Rosenthal staring directly into Bela's hazel eyes.

Without flinching Bela solemnly shook her head. Mrs Rosenthal repeated the question and Bela repeated the solemn shake. Losing patience Mrs Rosenthal said 'Why do you think that Louise and Sarah would waste my time with silly stories? Can you tell me because I really don't understand why they'd say they saw you putting it in your satchel last night, do you?'

Bela still did not speak. Slamming her silver Parker on the desk she repeated 'did you or did you not take that book?' Bela's heart thumped in her throat as she nodded slowly.

Mrs Rosenthal called Amit Bai and Mina at work. They turned up late. When they saw Bela's head hung low, and her absolute refusal to look them in the eye, they assumed the worst. Mrs Rosenthal gave Amit Bai and Mina a long boring spiel about the reprehensible nature of theft. She castigated them for not instilling ethical values in their daughter. Her shoddy appearance and sloppy homework was a reflection of tardiness in the home. Amit Bai wanted to give this supercilious bitch a good kick but for his daughter's sake he swallowed his anger in a single gulp. Mina disliked the insinuations. It was only a book. She had not committed a heinous crime. She hadn't killed anyone or tortured someone with bamboo sticks under nails she'd just stolen a book and now Bela faced possible expulsion. Bela received a warning, if she made one more mistake she was out.

Bela got the silent treatment on the bus home but as soon as Amit Bai and Mina entered the house the anger and shame spilt out like lumpy vomit over Bela. Amit Bai came out with a familiar stock of insults. A firm favourite of Mina's was 'Haramsada Kutha Saab' which in Bangla means, bastard son of a bitch followed by the classic line 'I wish you were never born'. Amit Bai ranted on 'Best bloody school in the country, bloody waste of money.'

And Bela momentarily lost her fear 'I never wanted to go to that bloody school anyway. I was doing OK at Amberleigh.'

Bela spat out a truckload of shit that had been festering inside her like a sceptic sore 'Why do you want me to be Number one? Why can't I be Number three hundred and twenty one? What's wrong with being thicker than a brick? You are not even my real father, you can't tell me what to do.'

Amit Bai told Bela to shut up but she refused. He suddenly struck out across Bela's left cheek. The skin began to sting, the tears started flowing and Bela embraced the smacks, the kicks and slaps with open arms because self-defence was out of the question. Amit Bai and Mina inflated into a pair of monumental fat columns. They appeared terrifying and awesome. In real life they were both diminutive and pear shaped. They loomed over Bela with flared nostrils and screwed up faces. Bela believed that if she cried loud enough they would leave her alone but the sobbing just aggravated them even more. Mina ordered Bela to 'stop crying and try to think about what you've done to us.'

Amit Bai was getting increasingly frustrated. He needed to find a way to gag the demons raving in Bela's head. Amit Bai dragged Bela by the arm to her room and flung Bela onto the bed. Her body curled into a foetal position. Amit Bai spotted two Danger Mouse dressing gowns hanging from the wardrobe. He removed the belts, held down Bela's feet, tied up her ankles, pulled her arms back and bound her wrists. Bela's body was contorted beyond recognition, her neck bent forwards, her shoulders forced back and her legs twisted. Amit Bai left her there on the bed and went downstairs for something to eat.

When Mrs Bond and Ana walked into the house and Amit Bai asked her to leave for the day she knew that something was not quite right. Amit Bai told Ana not to go into the bedroom but she sneaked in anyway because it was her room too. She saw her sister lying on the bed tied up in knots, talking to herself for comfort. Bela must have done something terrible to deserve this. She must have pushed Daddy to the edge because Daddy wouldn't have done this for any old thing. Ana wanted to reach out to her sister and hold her but already from an early age she found it difficult to receive a kiss from her parents or administer a hug so Ana stood there like a limp piece of lettuce unable to utter a word of consolation. After a minute or two of silent staring Ana left and returned with a stale bowl of popcorn that had been sitting by the bread bin for a week.

'Are you hungry?' Bela shook her head.

Ana smiled at her sister hoping that it would make her feel better but she didn't smile back. She just told her to 'Get out.'

Ana left and spotted Rimi doing her maths homework in the small room. Mina was busy watering her Ivy in the bathtub happily lost in her own world. Ana went downstairs and found Amit Bai in the kitchen reading the paper over a plate of chapattee, fried egg and leftover kebabs. Bela was still tied up in the bedroom and no one seemed that bothered. At ten o'clock Amit Bai went upstairs and finally untied her.

Bela found it hard to forgive and forget everything with a big hug. She refused to speak to her parents for two weeks after the ‘tying up’ incident; in fact she didn’t speak to anyone really. Ana would find Bela sat in her corner in front of the fan heater. She remained stubbornly mute at school, handed in her homework deliberately late with mandatory ink stains. She clung onto nasty memories and catalogued them in chronological order. Mummy might be nice one day, Daddy might make her giggle on another and they might feel closer than ever before but the memories of slaps and petty altercations lingered. Bela's meticulous mental catalogue was ammunition for the next confrontation and absolution for her naughtiness.

One quiet Saturday morning Mina was busily preparing a huge dinner. They were having six guests over that evening. There were still onions to slice, garlic to crush, fish to wash, prawns to peel, chicken to marinade, lentils to boil and rice to simmer. Mina was tired, her back was killing her, she needed to lie down and there was the washing waiting to be hung. She asked Bela to do it and went to bed for a quick nap.

Two hours later Mina woke up, realised the time and panicked. She ran downstairs to find an empty basket sitting by the sink and a leaden lump of washing lying in the belly of the machine. Bela was upstairs, reading her book, happily picking her toes, lost in a fantasy world of dark winding forests and strange phallic hills. Mina yelled at Bela to come down. Ten minutes later Bela appeared and Mina tried to poke an explanation out of the sulking child. Bela finally said 'I forgot.'

Annoyed by her nonchalance Mina screamed 'I'm not a bloody servant you know. I need help, not much, just a little. Go on, hang the clothes then.'

'It's not fair; the others are watching the A - Team.'Bela muttered.

Mina marched into the sitting room and shouted 'turn if off or I'll break that damn thing.' Rimi promptly turned off the TV. Ana was slightly annoyed because it had just reached the best part, where Mr T and the rest of the team construct an ingenious devise to confound the baddies.

Rimi started to cut onions and Ana did the washing up. Once Bela had hung the clothes she skulked off but Mina dragged her back into the kitchen, thrust a baseball bat in her hands and told her to 'crush garlic'. Bela stared at the four cloves huddled together in the big stone dish. She knew she ought to peel them carefully but she couldn't be bothered and, grabbing the bat, vented her anger on the four little cloves. Mina freaked out when she saw the uneven pulp. 'What are you doing? Give it to me. Go on go upstairs. You're bloody useless.'

Before Bela could run off Mina said 'you can polish my shoes instead.'

Bela saw the shoes on the landing. They were covered in a thick film of dust and hard mud. She pulled out a pot of polish, socks and brushes from an old Next bag. 'Remove excess dirt before applying polish' she read. It seemed too much like hard work. Bela filled the sink with hot water and flung the shoes in for a soak instead. Then she slumped onto her bed and continued to read her book. Chapter five lead to chapter six followed by seven. An hour later Bela returned to the shoes. They were drenched. Bela panicked and tried to dry them with a hair dryer. Mina was halfway up the stairs. Bela was still blow-drying. Seeing her beautiful Bally shoes, pale and discoloured Mina yelled 'what have you done? Do you know how expensive these shoes are?'

Mina picked up one of the shoes and chucked it at Bela. She ducked and the shoe landed in the bath next to the Ivy. Mina ran over to the plant and inspected the damage while Bela was slumped on the stairs rubbing her sore shoulder.

'Stay in your room and don't come out until I tell you to,' warned Mina

Bela locked herself in the bathroom and sat on the loo. Perhaps she should have hung up the washing and peeled the garlic. Perhaps she shouldn't have put Mummy's nice leather Bally shoes in the sink. Perhaps then she wouldn't get smacked and family life would be sweet. Bela didn't think she had done anything wrong, it was Mina who was in the wrong.

GUNGI BLUES

Hitting her over a silly pair of shoes. Who did she think she was? Mina didn't seem that bothered about her shoulder; she cared more about her stupid Ivy than her kids. Bela stared at the healthy green plant sitting smugly in the bath, basking in the light. Its stems flowed over the side like a green waterfall. Tiny baby leaves, almost transparent and furry with soft hairs, were beginning to unfold. They were everywhere. Delicate and tender. The Ivy was too big for the house now and Amit Bai urged Mina to sell it. He was positive they would get at least twenty quid for the plant without even trying. Mina refused. She remembered how it started off as a fragile cutting in a tiny pot. Over the years she watched it grow into the splendid mass it was today. The Ivy was her baby. It never answered back, never had mood swings; it just needed water and sun.

A pair of blunt rusty scissors lay by the sink. Mina used them to trim Amit Bai's moustache. Bela picked them up, walked calmly to the plant and brushed her hand along a flurry of baby leaves. Within a second she decapitated five stems in a single snip and the baby leaves fell one by one onto the bathroom mat. She could have settled for this. Mina would never have noticed but once she started she couldn't stop. The snip snip of the scissors continued faster and faster and her hand seemed to move by itself until all that remained was a sporadic sprouting of leaves in the middle. Bela hadn't intended to cut so much. If only she could Sellotape the one hundred stems back together.

She carefully replaced the scissors, retreated to bed and tried to lose herself in manufactured dreams.

Half an hour later Bela heard Mina's out of tune singing. She was changing out of her night dress into a red silk sari with a subtle purple border. Brushing her hair into a neat bun she added some blusher to her cheeks and a lacing of her new Estee Lauder lipstick. Elegant and beautiful she was ready to receive the guests and seduce their bellies with her gorgeous cooking. The plough was moist, the prawns tender, the chicken crisp, the aloo soft and the fish burning with red chillies. She ran into the bathroom to touch up her lips and at first she did not notice anything awry until she looked down and saw her toes submerged in green leaf. Mina wailed out. Bela heard the bedroom door open and Mina's cursing. She tried to protect her face with her arms but Mina's palms found her cheeks. Amit Bai walked through the front door, tired and hungry; he was not in the mood for any 'naughty giddy'. When Mina told him what 'that monster' had done he automatically ordered Bela to squat in the 'Murga' position. 'Murga' is a traditional punishment involving squatting, looping your arms behind your knees and clasping your ears. Within two minutes searing pain travels up your neck, your arms begin to ache and your legs cramp up. After five minutes of squatting in the pose Bela began to groan. Ana sat on the stairs and stared at her contorted lump of a sister. Bela told Ana to 'get lost'.

Ana replied with a slight grin, 'you shouldn't have cut up the plant Bela. That was very, very naughty of you.'

Bela told Ana to 'shut your gob'.

A fight was brewing and Ana could smell it. Soon they were screaming at one another. It was the usual - shut up you cow, get lost you pig - stuff. The squabble was enough to irritate Amit Bai and as punishment, he ordered Ana to twist her body into Murga.

It dawned on them how ridiculous they must have looked. Two malfongulated sisters clasping their ears. This wasn't a punishment it was some sick game conceived by a deranged Bengali woman. Every ten minutes Amit Bai checked that they were not relaxing the squat. Their legs were numb, arms aching, ears burning and still they squatted. To ease the pain they sang 'Johnny Briggs.' The doorbell rang and they jumped into the shadows. Amit Bai ran into the hallway to open the door. The first guest was Uncle Mumtaz. His second hand, champagne gold Datsun was parked outside and Amit Bai said 'nice car.'

Uncle Mumtaz spotted Bela and Ana lurking in a dark corner and grabbing Ana's head with his hand he thumped it with the other, then he sauntered into the kitchen. Mina looked on passively as he dipped his wrinkled finger into the coconut prawn curry, scooped up a prawn and chomped it down. Despite the fact that all his food tasted of tomato ketchup, he fancied himself as a bit of a gourmet cook and always insisted on sampling everything. Bela and Ana watched with a mixture of disgust and envy. They would have got a good slap for nibbling on prawns but Uncle Mumtaz could do as he pleased. The guests dripped in one by one. There was Uncle Saleem who never changed his socks; Uncle Dilip who said 'Jesus Christ' every other minute; Uncle Farhan with the creepy eyes; and then there were the wives. Auntie Saleem was small with a hamster like face and glasses that consumed half her face. Uncle Mumtaz's wife was freshly plucked from Bangladesh. She expected red carpets and washing machines, not pubic hairs on the toilet seat when she arrived in England. 'Why do we drive a second hand Datsun and Amit Bai drives a Sierra?' She complained. Still she dutifully produced a son and was four months pregnant with another kid. Auntie Farhan always carried fragments of tissue for her permanently blocked sinuses. Her daughters', Farhana and Cuckoo, both had the same nasal affliction. When the three of them sat together the sound of blowing noses filled their ears. Finally, there was Aunty Dilip. She used to have a perm and was rather glamorous but after she got married she became an over weight slap head.

Mina offered a constant flow of Coca Cola, Tetley's tea and Chana Chor. No one would have suspected that she was bereaving her beloved Ivy.

For now they were playing happy, perfect families in that little house. The house creaked under the burden of so many people. The three-piece suite could only seat five small bums, six if you were lucky. People sat on the edge of chairs and the floor. The air was thick with chatter. Ana couldn't hear herself think and observed their lovely guests with curiosity. Uncle Saleem was wriggling his toes and Uncle Mumtaz was rubbing the dry skin from behind his ears. Both were talking to one another but neither was really listening to what the other was saying. Amit Bai tended to the wives, patiently listening to everything from financial worries to the state of their kids' teeth. When Mina announced that dinner was ready people filed into the living room and within minutes there were gravy splatters on the lace tablecloth and rice on the carpet. Uncle Mumtaz allowed dhal to dribble down the side of his mouth and Uncle Saleem picked his teeth. All that mattered was the food. People spoke with full mouths, belched in one another's faces and Ana watched nimble fingers produce perfect balls of rice and plates swept clean with palms. Once the food was devoured there were still the bones. A frenetic chomping session ensued until all that remained were purple mounds on plates. With his four teeth Amit Bai sucked on his bone like a baby's dummy. Dinner was over. Bela and Ana cleared the table. She washed, Ana dried up and Uncle Mumtaz rubbed his tooth on a purple towel as he tried to dislodge the fleck of meat stuck between his front two teeth. The family used that towel to wipe their hands and faces. Bela and Ana wanted to smash his face in but settled for violent nostril flaring instead. Uncle Mumtaz didn't seem to notice the nostrils, asked Ana to make him 'tea with two sugars and milk' and left.

For desert Mina had made a Birds Eye Trifle from a packet. The white fluffy cream of the trifle looked like cloud. It was a shame to shatter the illusion with hundreds and thousands. Mina scolded Bela for taking out the red plastic bowls instead of the posh ones from Kendals. Apart from Mina, Bela didn't think anyone would have noticed the plastic from the porcelain. The guests were too busy gorging on sweet things and cups of cha. Ana sat opposite Uncle Farhan's daughter, enjoying the red jelly in the trifle. As she talked something catapulted from her mouth and landed in the corner of Ana's eye. It felt cold and wet. Felt like she'd been assaulted. Ana wanted them all to piss off back home now. No one budged an inch even though the conversation was drying up and no one found Uncle Mumtaz's jokes funny. Mina dimmed the lights and decided to put on a bud bud movie. Although Bela and Ana didn't understand the Hindi they liked the bright colours, the guaranteed wet sari scenes, the dancing in the bush and the ting ting of the songs. The plots never seemed to change in bud bud movies. There was always a man in white jeans and a pink shirt from a poor family who fancies Dimple, the rich Daddy's girl, who is lonely and unhappy. By chance Dimple and Pink Jeans meet on a hill and fall desperately in love but there is a rich baddy, with a seriously deep voice and sweaty face who wants to unravel Dimple's sari and bite her belly button. An inevitable confrontation ensues in a dark alleyway and Pink Jeans gets beaten up, loses his job and ends up without the girl and on the streets. They have a secret rendezvous at a Hindu temple and suddenly it starts to rain. Her sari becomes all wet and clingy as she hides coquettishly behind a tree, shakes her hips and sings a beautiful love song in a shrill, nasal voice. They disappear in the long grass and suddenly it's morning and you know they have done jiggy jiggy. We soon discover that Sweaty Face is embezzling money from Dimple's gullible father and ironically Dimple's Daddy thinks the sun shines out of Sweaty Face's arse. Pink Jeans tries to tell Dimple's Daddy that Sweaty Face is screwing him over. Dimple's Daddy is not having any of it but checks his accounts anyway. When he smells a rotten fish he confronts Sweaty Face and suddenly Sweaty Face draws out a machete from his underpants and threatens to kill him if he doesn't hand over everything including his daughter. Dimple and Pink Jeans walk in and a fast and furious bloody fight begins along with a singsong and a thunderstorm. Another fifty baddies appear from nowhere, start doing a very cool synchronised dance and break out in song. Pink Jeans manages to kill all of them and finally stabs Sweaty Face in the tummy. Dimple starts crying with joy. Dimple's Daddy hugs Pink Jeans and Dimple and Pink Jeans get hitched. The End.

At three o'clock in the morning people finally started to leave. Ana never understood why their parents bothered entertaining at all. She didn't think they really connected with these people, it was a hassle cooking for so many and the house was always trashed by the end of the evening. Uncle Mumtaz and his wife were the last to leave. His wife tried to talk to Ana in Bangla and she shied away in embarrassment. They knew how to say, dog shit is very hot, their numbers from one to ten, cunt, bastard, son of a bitch, bless you, hello, good-bye, rice, goat, frog and mango but that was about it. Uncle Mumtaz's two-year-old son knew more Bangla than Bela and Ana put together. Unable to help himself, he castigated Mina for failing to teach her children Bangla and then implored her to 'come to my house Babi. Please come Babi.' before driving off into the night in his flash Datsun. Mina closed the door and looked slightly disgruntled

'It's embarrassing that you lot don't speak Bangla. Speak Bangla. Go on,' she said

'Why do you always speak to them in English, that's why they can't speak the language.' Mina complained to Amit Bai.

Amit Bai joined in for the sake of it 'Listen to your mother, go on speak Bangla.' The children groaned as their parents' nagged them incessantly.

If they were honest they listened to Duran Duran more than Runa La La, at school Rimi learned about William Shakespeare not Rabindranath Tagore and they seemed to prefer the Peter's to the Mohammed's at school. They were not total Bounty bars. Ana and her sisters ate dhal and rice with their hands, used a jug and bowl to wash with, ate green chillies, were quite partial to a bowl of Roshaguli and liked to listen to Mina's Pakeezah album. Ana particularly liked the soothing solo flute bits. In some ways they were Bengali, in others English but in essence they were neither. They were Banglish, a strange blend, a curious hybrid, a hotch potch.

It seemed rather late in the day to start teaching them Bangla but it didn't stop Mina from buying a heap of Bangla books. The following Sunday she tried to make them sit down for an hour and learn 'Kor, Khor, Gor, Ghor.' Rimi made more progress than Bela and Ana. They never really got beyond the 'I like mango' stage. It didn't help that Mina fell asleep after half an hour. It wasn't just the poor Bangla that bothered her. Her children were born Muslim and none of them knew how to practise the faith. They didn't eat pig or drink booze, well Amit Bai had the occasional beer in the pub to keep his work mates happy and Mina liked the taste of Whiskey when she had a cold. Amit Bai and Mina didn't didn't pray five times a day, they only pulled the prayer mats out when there was a crisis. Ana had been to the Mosque but it was only for weddings. The Mosque was a shabby hall just off the curry mile in Rusholme. At the weddings Ana attended she remembered seeing kids playing hide and seek under the tables and people dishing food out of buckets.

Worried that her children would end up culturally barren and completely Westernised, Mina employed an Uzur to come to the house every Friday to teach Arabic and the Holy Koran. The Uzur was tall, with a long silver beard and no moustache. His eyes were black with fierce bushy eyebrows locked in a permanent frown that severed his forehead in two. His expression was grim, his thin lips were pursed and unused to smiling. One cheek bulged with a pocket of Paan and his red stained teeth made him look like a cannibal. He inspected the living room and looked disapprovingly at the paintings on the wall. He insisted on removing a nude wooden carving and a few landscapes. Then he asked Mina for a white sheet to cover the floor. Dressed casually in jeans and jumpers the old man told Ana to 'get changed' and enquired 'Have you done Namaz?'

Namaz was the mandatory ritualistic wash performed by Muslims before prayer. It felt odd washing her feet in the sink five times over. Ana did the same with her hands, arms, ears and face, whispering Bismallah Hirach Man Nir A Hime, not knowing what it meant. When Ana entered the sitting room door all their belongings were concealed under a stretch of white. The Uzur sat cross-legged on the floor and handed them each a thin, grey book. The front cover was covered in Arabic and Ana followed the elegant curls and shapes of the letters as they danced along the page. The Uzur opened the book and began to recite the letters: 'Alif, bey, tey. sey...' They watched and listened then he grunted at them to repeat the letters.

The letter 'Ghaarff' became their favourite. A deep guttural sound produced from the back of the throat like a burp gone slightly wrong. For two hours they repeated the rhythmic sounds, gently rocking back and forth. The Uzur just sat and listened, pouncing on them when they made a mistake.

The novelty wore off and they began to dread Fridays. They were just reciting a bunch of strange letters, which had no meaning to them. Amit Bai and Mina refused to give up after only two weeks and bought their own personal hard back covered Korans for each child. Ana genuinely wanted to read the Holy book but she gave up after the first ten pages because she didn't understand it. The exercise into religion and Bangla was not totally futile; Bela and Ana did manage to memorise two prayers 'Bismillah Hirack Man Nirahim ... ' and 'Kul Hu Wallah Hu Wahad ... ' from an 'Easy learn guide' poster Mina purchased from a shop in Rusholme. Although Ana's pronunciation was crap she used to compete with Bela to see who could recite the prayers the fastest. To them they were just funny sounds that tickled their palettes and after a few weeks quickly forgotten. They never really grasped what the Muslim faith was all about. All they knew was that they couldn't eat pig because it was a dirty, filthy animal that ate its own shit and alcohol was an evil poison that made your breath smell. And when Ana asked Mina 'What does it mean to be a good Muslim?' she replied 'To be a good person, that's being a good Muslim.'

Amit Bai and Mina decided to cancel their Friday lessons with the Uzur because they were going to Bangladesh over Christmas. The three children had never been before. Their parents never told them why they were going. Perhaps Mina missed her folks. Perhaps Amit Bai thought it was about time that his folks met his new wife and kids. Perhaps for the first time they had saved enough money to afford the trip. Or perhaps they just wanted to show them where they really came from, wherever that was.

Ana accompanied Amit Bai to the mosque to break the news to the Uzur. When they arrived, Amit Bai told Ana to wait for him in the other room while he did Namaz. That's when Ana noticed how all the men were assembled in the prayer hall and the women in another. The men performed Namaz with synchronised precision. Amit Bai was one of those kneeling, muttering, bending men and it seemed totally incongruous seeing him pray. Ana listened to the sound of prayer, deep and melodic. The Uzur was standing on the podium reciting prayer with rhythmic perfection. His face was deadly serious and there was an odour of solemnity and socks in the air. After Namaz, the Uzur was swallowed up in a crowd of black and white bearded men. Amit Bai and Ana looked for a while but there was no trace of him. His house was not far. The Uzur lived on a row of semi detached, shoebox, red brick houses just off Wilmslow Road. Amit Bai decided to pay him a visit. When they reached the Uzur's house, Amit Bai paused as the sound of screaming and shouting pierced the walls. Amit Bai waited for the fight to subside. It just seemed to intensify so he knocked anyway and a little boy answered the door. He was skinny and barefooted. Ana looked in and saw a house, similar to their own, with splintering skirting boards and cracks in the wall. The Uzur appeared in a lungi and white T Shirt looking slightly small and crumpled. Amit Bai politely said 'we won't need you to teach the children anymore because we are going to Bangladesh in December. When we get back we'll call you.'

The Uzur listened to Amit Bai in silence and then shut the door. As Ana and Amit Bai walked down the street they heard the sound of shouting once more. Without his furry grey hat, his garb, his podium and Koran the Uzur was not an awesome paragon of religion, he was just an ordinary man.

Ana's flirtation with religion was over and from then on she became agnostic.

Sanchita Islam

A Bit of Bangladesh

It was a week before their trip to Bangladesh. Amit Bai and Mina bought bags of gifts: paint boxes, sketchbooks, Rubik's Cubes, M&S bras and Quality Street chocolates. It felt like Christmas but none of it was for them apart from the twenty packets of Cup-a-Soup, four tubs of Horlicks and three boxes of Sugar Puffs. It was a precaution, just in case the food over there didn't agree with the children. It seemed like they were going away for six months not four weeks. In total they packed five cases and then there were all the tiny plastic bags too.

The day had finally arrived. They crammed into a taxi on a chilly Saturday morning. Amit Bai's knees were brimming over with bags 'Why did you bring so much stuff?' he snapped at Mina.

Mina ignored him but then she didn't have to carry any of it. Between the three sisters they carried nine bags.

There was no hassle at Manchester airport. It was like hopping onto the 172 bus to school. Heathrow, by contrast, was mayhem with queues of people, crying babies, silver trolleys, nasal voices and excess baggage. They queued to check in their luggage and Ana stared at the chocolate skins, dark eyes and jet-black oiled hair of other Bangladeshis. Ana felt like a minority within a minority. Mutually suspicious, like Man U and Liverpool fans, they tried to suss one another out.

GUNGI BLUES

These were her fellow compatriots, her brown brothers and sisters but Ana was uncomfortable. Bombarded by the sound of chatter, strange smells, red stained lips and staring eyes, Ana pined for a silent, spacious moment. It never came. When it was time to board, people leapt up, pushing their way onto the plane, as if they feared it would take off without them. Ana was flying for the first time and she envisaged plush fittings, wide aisles and capacious seats. When she boarded the plane Ana saw worn out seating and thin carpets, sticky underfoot. She sat down and the man sitting adjacent to her started to rub his well-worn toes. Ana looked away and noticed a sucked lemon rind, a blackcurrant boiled sweet and a used tissue lying in the aisle way.

They prepared to take off and Ana gripped the sides of her seat as she felt her belly rise into her mouth and her ears pop. Looking down through the snippets of cloud Ana gazed at London, a place she had not yet explored. Thousands of lights lit up the city and it looked like an amazing, flash place. Ana prodded Bela to take a look but she just pulled a face and thumped her. Ana tried to play eye spy by herself. She tried to sleep but ended up watching restless men patrol the aisles bare foot. It didn't concern them that they were causing an obstruction. She observed faces darkened from too many days in the blaring sun and pitted skin ravaged by hungry mosquitoes. Ana saw moustached men in patterned tops, Bill Cosby style jumpers, baggy jackets, white cotton shirts, trainers and sandals. And two women dressed in patterned purple, puffy shouldered, flower print dresses and black-heeled shoes decorated in gold. The air on the plane was clogged up with spice, dust and sweat. It was hard to sleep. Ana tried, only to be woken up by a strange and vigorous sound. She opened her eyes to see a man with his leg cocked on the armrest with his trouser pulled up to the knee. He was itching his calf. Ana closed her eyes again, stuck on a pair of headphones, tuned into channel three and let Duran Duran blast in her ears for a while. Then a Bollywood movie kept Ana entertained with its ridiculous plot, its jiggling about on the street, its men in tight trousers and its pouting big-eyed stars. Ana couldn't concentrate on the film because the man sitting adjacent to her wouldn't stay still. He looked around every few minutes, eyes bloodshot, searching for something. Those eyes kept her awake until the black of night disintegrated into orange, green, yellow and purple. Bullets of bleached out light shot through the portholes and clouds drifted like smoke across a stretch of blue and it looked like heaven.

At 4 am the multi ethnic airhostesses offered light breakfast. Most passengers abstained because it was the month of Ramadan: the holy month of prayer and dedicated fasting from first light to sunset. Ana felt almost guilty drinking the orange juice on offer but she drank it anyway.

There was one hour to landing. Snoozing, Ana held a pen loosely in her left hand. The man sitting adjacent to her took it. He didn't ask he just took it, used it, and then returned it. Fifteen minutes to landing. Ana arched her neck for a glimpse of a bit of Bangladesh. She saw that others were excited like her. Excited to see the 'Desh'. Through a murky mist the land emerged. A Mondrian grid of curved out shapes and green. Ana saw the reflection of trees in the brown still water. It resembled a monumental abstract painting of endless lines, squares, rectangles and delicate forms. They landed with a bump and the runway was surrounded by overgrown grass that stretched out into a band of trees and bush. They could have been in the jungle. The plane was moving and the seatbelt sign flashing but people leapt out of their seats desperate to get off the plane. The airhostesses sighed as they observed the crushing chaos. Amit Bai told the children to stay put and they were one of the last to disembark. As they emerged from the plane a brilliant white light made them squint and look down. It was a stark contrast to the drizzle, wind and cold of Manchester. Clouds of dust wafted up their nose and the runway was dotted with dark brown faces and stick thin legs. They filed into the airport with a pile of crumpled others. Enormous luminous 'No Smoking' signs hung from the ceiling. 'Smoking, littering and chewing gum strictly prohibited' Ana quickly swallowed her Wrigley's gum and when she looked out the large windows she saw gigantic toothpicks arranged in tubes. There were scores of them and Ana had no clue what they were.

A long line of people gathered at passport control. There were two booths: one was for Bangladeshi nationals, the other for non-nationals. The men sitting behind the booths seemed in no immediate hurry. One man was reading his paper, the other digging into his nose and the third slowly checking each passport. In the distance a man stood by a makeshift desk. 'PLANT QUARANTINE: Any plants, fruits, spices or plant stuff to be checked here please' read the sign. After wrestling with a stubborn trolley Amit Bai guided them over to the conveyor belt. It was swarming with nervous looking folk. A man appeared on the conveyor belt, but there was still no luggage. She stared up at the metallic ceiling to kill time. A podgy fair skinned woman standing with her small son, dressed in a shiny brown suit, complained 'Why is it taking so long?' And then large cases padded up in bright torn quilts and plastic bottles of leaking water, started to chug by. Fifteen minutes later the cases arrived and they could go.

Ana saw masses of people waiting outside, pressed up against bars, looking out for familiar faces. She hoped someone was looking out for them too. Amit Bai pushed their trolley past those staring eyes. There were people everywhere, stretching out way beyond the airport. An old man with white stubble that shone against his black skin tried to help Amit Bai. He seemed weak and frail. On his last legs. But he still carried cases on his back. Ana saw a couple of ladies wearing beige ribbed polo necks, gold bangles and red lipstick.

GUNGI BLUES

They were bickering loudly, entertaining passersby. A kid, barefoot and spindly, tugged at one lady's sleeve. She told the kid to 'get lost' in Bangla and shooed him away with a hand but the kid didn't seem bothered. Amit Bai and Mina scanned the crowd. A tall figure, dressed in military uniform with shoes so shiny they glowed, was combing his shoe polish black dyed hair. He was looking in their direction and after putting away his comb he walked towards them. 'Amit Bai' he boomed slapping him on the back.

'Babi how are you?' He said looking Mina up and down.

He was Mezu Kalu, Mina's brother in law. He had married Conna. With a few clicks of his finger they bypassed disgruntled passengers and were escorted to three white cars. They piled into the cars and slowly left the bustle. The heat was crawling up Ana's skin. She needed a bath and clean bed. She'd been travelling too long. Sitting in the car Ana looked out the window and tried to take it all in. The eaten up roads, the piles of dirt on the sidewalk, the lush green trees, the half naked kids carrying half empty bottles of water and bulging sacks. Ana opened her ears to let in the sounds. The sound of car horns, the tinkle tinkle of bells, the beep beep of impatient drivers and the underlying crackle that refused to die.

They drove down wide dusty roads dotted with rickshaw drivers, baby taxis, hand painted bill boards and rickety buildings and entered a leafy suburb lined with tall Deb Daru trees and white washed walls. This was Gulshan, the affluent part of Dhaka, where people with money lived in relative luxury with their two point three servants. They reached tall iron gates manned by two guards carrying rifles on their shoulders. The guards saluted Mezu Kalu and raced to see who could open the gates first. Ana looked out the window and saw a massive white house, marble stairs, a thick wooden door and bursts of red flowers. Rimi was dumb struck but Bela seemed indifferent. As Ana fumbled with the car door a servant stepped forward and calmly opened it. Ana and her sisters dribbled out the car and huddled together on the marble stairs feeling out of place. Their parents were too engrossed in conversation with Mezu Kalu and ignored them. Ana caught the odd word in Bangla and gave up after ten seconds. They were simply talking too quickly. Mezu Kalu walked into the house and led them into the living room. A vast room with red sofas, red patterned carpet and a cheap chandelier. A tallish lady with fair skin draped in an elegant blue sari walked in. It was Mina's sister Conna Kala. She had all the same features, high cheekbones, button nose, big eyes and fat lips with glasses that were far too big for her face. Although Conna Kala and Mina hadn't seen one another for years there was no hug, just an exchange of insipid smiles. She glanced down at the three children and said ‘they are so thin.’

Mina replied defensively 'It was a long flight. They are tired and haven't eaten.'

As Ana watched Conna, the stories Mina told them came flooding back. Conna was the one who was forced to lie on a table while Nanu pulled a worm out of her bum. She was the one who bought chocolates with money stolen from Nana's pot and pretended they were a gift from a passing stranger on the street. She was the one who, for no apparent reason, pulled a knife on Mina and slashed her stomach. She was the one who was always getting beaten with a stick of sugar cane for some naughty deed when she was a kid. Now Conna sat serene and still. A pair of large tinted glasses dominated her face. Her arms were bare, white and hairless. She leant forward, turned on the TV and quickly became engrossed. Mezu Kala told them that he had to do Namaz and would be back in ten minutes or so. They were left sitting in the living room watching a drama where the actresses were caked in too much make up speaking a language Ana and her sisters didn't understand. Mezu Kalu re-animated the room with his return. In his arms he carried a photo album and proudly showed them photographs of himself standing next to the President of Bangladesh, General Zia. Then he showed them a double spread devoted to photos of a plot of land.

'I am building a four story house so that I can have a flat for each of my children.' He said proudly. 'One day Shofkot will be a Lieutenant, he's only four now and. Rafat's doing very well. His teachers all say he's a brilliant student.'

Amit Bai and Mina listened intently. Rimi, pretending that she understood the Bangla when she didn't really. Bela and Ana fidgeted with boredom, pulling at their winter jumpers that were sticky with sweat. Something caught Bela's eye. 'Did you see that?' she hissed. Ana looked up to see a lizard crawl out a crack and a shy face watched them from behind the door. She flashed a smile of Colgate white teeth and beckoned Bela and Ana with her tiny hand. Curious, they approached the skinny girl.

The girl's name was Alice, as in Alice in Wonderland, but she pronounced it Ellis. Ellis was Conna Kala's daughter. She took Bela and Ana to a bedroom with a King sized bed and a Hi Fi, and produced an array of Beatles records from under the bed. They were soon bouncing up and down on the bed, singing 'It's been a hard day's night.' Conna came in after ten minutes and told them to stop jumping up and down like 'pagulls'. Watching Conna castigate Ellis with her shrill voice and raised fist was uncannily familiar. When Conna left, Ellis's dazzling grin reappeared and she took Bela and Ana outside into the brilliant sun. The garden was squashed with tall slender trees bearing puny round green apples. Like a monkey, Ellis climbed up the tree and began to shake it until the green apples fell to the ground. Ana picked one up and examined the strange thing. Ellis jumped down from the tree and landed in a froggy position. She scoured the ground, discarding several before selecting the perfect green thing and offered it to Ana. She called it 'borrowee' and said it was 'kup moza,' Out of politeness Ana took a bite and her teeth met a stone. The taste was bitter but sweet, the flesh hard but soft. Ellis told them to wait a minute. She darted back into the house and returned with a bowl swimming with green chilli, oil and lemon juice. Ana dipped one borrowee into the mixture and then stuffed it into her mouth. Although her tongue burned and her eyes watered Ana continued to eat. An hour later, Bela and Ana lay next to a small heap of borrowee stones. Groaning as their stomachs churned, Ellis was still munching away. Conna discovered them lying on the grass clutching their bellies. She swiped the dish of chilli oil from Ellis's hands and told them to 'go inside and wash your hands. Dinner's ready.'

'We're not hungry' Bela whined.

'Come on' said Conna in a tone they thought best not to disobey.

Bela and Ana followed Ellis as she skipped to the dining room and a feast of fish, prawns, spicy salad, chicken and watermelon was waiting for them. Ellis attacked the food on the table while Bela and Ana picked at it. The rice tasted weird and the chicken legs were puny and tough. Only the spicy salad tasted good and with each mouthful their stomachs protested loudly.

After dinner Conna showed them to their room. It was spacious with one double bed, a desk, a bookshelf and drawn curtains that made the room much too dark.

That night Bela and Ana lay awake under the net fearful of the strange sounds. A tiny lizard kept them company but they wanted it to go away. They didn't turn off the light because they were afraid to be alone in the dark. It was a sleepless night in an alien land. Hot and sticky, they tossed and turned. Must be eight at least Ana thought. She looked at her watch. It was early morning and the whole of Bangladesh was united in prayer. Thousands of voices echoed through loud speakers. An incredible wailing, chanting sound that penetrated deep. The sound subsided to be replaced with a cock, cock cocking, a motorbike rev, the odd beep, occasional chirp and the mutter of voices.

Ana and Bela both refused to go to the bathroom because they were positive a cockroach was lying in wait for them. They heard the buzzing of frustrated mosquitoes that clung to the net waiting for blood. Bela and Ana whacked them with pillows and smothered their bodies with repellent that repelled them with its stink. Then they hid under white sheets and tried to sleep. It was impossible. Their bladders and bowels refused to give them peace and after ten minutes Bela whispered 'I need a wee.' Ana needed to go too but the thought of monster cockroaches was too scary to contemplate.

'Let's wait 'til morning. Try and sleep.'

'I can't. Please come with me. I can't go on my own,' Bela sounded desperate

'Think of sheep or something,' Ana whispered back.

Ana drifted off. She felt a warm stream travel down her legs. Smooth and lovely, she didn't want that stream to end but then it very quickly turned cold and left Ana stuck to the sheets. The following morning they heard footsteps and the sound of the net being pulled down. Bela and Ana pretended to be asleep. A cold breeze hit their legs as the sheets were whipped away. Conna muttered something in Bangla and returned with Mina.

'How could you wet the bed?' Mina yelled. Conna looked on with cool eyes. They didn't bother explaining about the monster cockroaches and giant mosquitoes; Mina and Amit Bai wouldn't understand.

Horses, Sprite and Sugar Puffs

Ana and Bela lay in bed for a little while. Ana was drawn to the snippets of clear blue sky that shone through the holes in the curtains. It was those snippets that enticed them out through a side door that led to the roof. They climbed up the ladder propped against the wall in their socks. Three crows swooped down on the ledge but they continued to climb. A leaking tank sat on the roof with a pool of green gunge beneath it. Autumn leaves somehow ended up there and the walls were discoloured and flaked into abstract shapes.

Ana looked up to see white washed walls, dancing trousers hanging from make shift clothes lines and the silhouettes of men on ledges, hammering away. Against this backdrop of activity, one man stood still. Uncontaminated by any sense of urgency, he just watched the others hard at work. Thick green foliage caressed the white flat top buildings. Palms nodded their leafy heads and Ana watched the rickshaws, the odd passer-by and the baby taxis speed past. Charmed by the plant pots, homes on sticks, pockets of water, its bang and caw caw, Ana and Bela stayed up on the roof until Conna's call for breakfast forced them down.

They sat at the table. A plate of chapattee, spicy potato and glasses of water were laid out. 'Can I have Sugar Puffs?' Bela requested.

A servant returned with a generous bowl of Puffs. Her name was Alu. Her hair was oiled black, her frame petite, her feet bare, her skin deep sepia. She was always doing something, if not cleaning the toilet, dusting under the table, or chopping downstairs. At night she slept on the floor in the living room. She didn't have a bed. She just hung a net from four corners of the room and lay down on some thin bedding. She was the first to wake and the last to sleep. She didn't complain, it was her job to serve, her job to be bossed, ordered and shouted at.

After breakfast they went back to their room. It was so dark and gloomy. All the curtains were drawn and Ana couldn't understand why knowing that there was a clear blue sky outside. Spread out in star shapes Ana and Bela felt the fans breathe on them. Then they went outside in the heat. Standing in the back garden weighed down with shiny saddles and brass trimmings were two horses. And all pressed and gleaming was Mezu Kalu sitting on one of them. Sweat ran like rivers down his beaming face as he combed his hair into place.

'Stand in front of the horse and let the photographer take your picture' he ordered.

For two hours Bela and Ana stood in blazing heat posing next to horses as they tried to eat grass. Mezu Kalu looked ridiculous with his medals, his garb, and his grin. Ana and Bela stood patiently, smiled and said thank you very much.

After the horse ordeal they were chauffeur driven to Mezu Kalu's cousin's house. They only lived up the road but no one really walked in Dhaka, there were no pavements to walk on. The house was shabby, run down with a patch of grass out front. They entered the house. The walls were crammed with romantic Bangladesh landscapes of boats sitting on tranquil waters and silent, lonely, riverbeds. Ana looked at the paintings closely. Do these pockets of quiet exist, she thought? Where were they? She hadn't seen them.

They sat in the living room, spacious and cool. Noticed that the paint on the wall was peeling from too many sweltering summers and the damp of the rains. The men in the room had bald patches and slightly round bellies, like Amit Bai. They spoke in Bangla and laughed riotously at jokes Ana didn't get. A young woman and man sat opposite, eyeing up Bela and Ana. The man had a face like a dog and a voice like a bark, the woman a sallow complexion and lank hair. 'Do you like my paintings?' She asked

Rimi was polite and said 'yes very much.' Bela and Ana made no comment.

'That's my father and mother. They were first cousins and got married when they were sixteen.' Said the young man.

Handsome and fresh in the photograph his parents were unrecognisable now. His mother was grossly over weight and his father flabby round the edges with thinning grey hair.

'My father used to work for the World Bank. He's travelled all over the world, but his health is not so good now.'

His sister butted in and said excitedly 'did you know that your father is my father's cousin? That makes us cousins!'

'You live in Manchester don't you? I used to live in Dallas. I worked there. I could have got American citizenship but Bangladesh is my home.' Babul waffled on.

'What do you do now?' Asked Rimi out of politeness.

'I work in the garments industry. I was studying medicine. I studied for two years. I've got the books, I can show you if you like. I'm practically a doctor but I gave it up. I got too scared; I don't like blood you see. Now I import and export garments. I have a shop in Dhaka, only embassy people come to my shop, I'll take you there if you like.'

'Do you live at home with your parents?' Asked Rimi.

Babul looked slightly uncomfortable. 'Most children live at home in Dhaka. There's no reason not to. My father has made me a little flat just out there. It's one room. Perfect for my wife and me.'

'That's nice.' Said Rimi running out of things to talk about.

A woman walked in, dressed in black. Her face was covered in spots, her skin blotchy and her hands and feet wrinkled like a little old lady.

'Babul' she said anxiously. 'Where's my counter?'

Babul produced the counter from his pocket; the woman grabbed it from his hand then she sat and click, click, clicked.

'You must excuse Lysu, my wife; she's depressed. Her father just died, she's usually so jolly.' Babul said.

Bela watched Lysu click the counter as she muttered under her breath.

'What are you doing?' Asked Bela

'I have to say Allah's name 50,000 times so that my father will go to heaven and rest in peace.'

Babul looked at his wife and said 'Why don't you do that later we're going to eat now?'

Lysu ignored her husband. Babul rolled his eyes. He forgot that there were people in the room and tried to grab the counter from Lysu's hands but she clenched her fist tight.

'Give it to me.' Babul was a huge brick of a man compared to his wife.

Lysu looked up from under her black veil and said calmly. 'You won't let me cry for my father's death, you won't let me talk to my friends, just let me do this?'

Babul turned to his sister 'do you see what I have to put up with?' His sister nodded sympathetically.

Lysu kept her eyes focused on her wrinkled fingers. Rimi began to fidget in discomfort.

'I'm going to check on Amma, Lysu are you coming with us?'

Lysu didn't answer so Babul and his sister left the room, leaving the three children alone with his wife. She stopped counting and stared at a wedding photo of her and Babul nailed to the wall.

'I used to look like a Barbie doll,' she said

'I used to be so fair. Look at me now. I'm only twenty six and my skin's dark and old like a Bura.'

'It must have been hard to lose your father,' said Rimi softly.

'He was my friend. Now I have no one. Babul just shouts at me. They all shout in this family, Babul's mother, father and sister. That's why I'm like this.' Lysu looked away and resumed her counting.

Babul's mother seemed like a rotund, smiling creature, his father weak with age, his sister a little strange and Babul too highly strung. Perhaps this lunch was a carefully planned show to make everyone think they were normal. Mina and Amit Bai did it all the time. Laughed at jokes that weren't very funny and shook hands with people they'd rather not.

Babul walked back in the room. There was paranoia in his eyes, he glared at his wife and said 'dinner's ready.'

A spread of dhal, kodhu, spinach, lamb, chicken, fish, aloo rice, salad and Sprite covered the table. Ana never much cared for Sprite but for some reason Babul's permanently smiling mother, dressed in bright yellow sari and large glasses, insisted that Ana drink Sprite. Everyone ate with his or her hands apart from Bela and Ana who preferred a knife and fork. Ana watched people deconstruct lamb, bite into long green chillies and add mango pickle for extra kick. Lysu picked at her food, hiding her face behind her black veil. Babul mashed banana with rice. He was on a diet. Trying to lose weight.

'Can you eat this food?' Babul's mother asked topping Ana's glass with more Sprite.

'Of course, I eat chillies everyday,' she laughed at her and Ana felt slightly sad.

Did they seem so English to them? Ana looked at her sisters. They stuck out in their green velvet pants, dungarees and flower patterned hats. No one talked to them at dinner, not even Mina or Amit Bai. They ate the greasy meat, oily rice, dry cucumber, drank too much Sprite and waited to go home,

Chickens and Whisky

It was early evening in Dhaka. The air smelt of sickness, cold and dust. Mina, Amit Bai and the kids were squeezed in a baby taxi because Mezu Kalu could not lend them his car. Ana and Bela sat on Amit Bai's knee and Bela balanced precariously on Mina's. The driver's head was wrapped tightly in a pink scarf and his shirt was full of holes. Ana tried to work out shadowy buildings dressed in waterfalls of fairy lights and wondered why there were so many Coca Cola signs. Ana was drawn to a massive billboard of a beautiful girl. She smiled down at the lady living in a shantytown on the other side of the road. The lady was adjusting her sari. She didn't wear a blouse. A limbless man slid past with his belly face down on a skateboard. He spotted a man with a paunch and squirrel red hair: 'Ek Takka' he begged but the man was too busy hailing a baby taxi.

They travelled to Dhanmondi where Attia, Amit Bai's cousin lived on the top floor of a block of flats. She had a balcony where you could see long lines of washing, buildings painted in red dots, bamboo sticks and cool verandas. The view was so thick with detail that Ana lost herself in windows and walls.

Attia, was bespectacled, short, with shoulder length hair. She spoke English with a creamy accent and took them downstairs to see her mother who lived on the ground floor. The old lady had kind eyes and a warm chuckle. She didn't say much, just smiled and nodded. Her back yard was full of plants and the occasional chicken. Almost like a farm but without the cows. Attia took them back upstairs. A skinny man sat in the corner with two teenagers dressed in T Shirts and jeans. There was half a bottle of Whisky on the table, which the skinny man was drinking neat. Seeing Amit Bai he leapt up and flung his arms around him like an old friend.

'Tariq Bai, how are you?' said Amit Bai with a huge grin.

'So so, things could be better.'

'What about Melia?' Tariq tensed up

'Melia's in the States.'

Tariq quickly stooped down, kissed the three children on both cheeks and introduced Ana and her sisters to his children, Misha and Tushki.

'Are you still living in Gulshan?' Asked Amit Bai

'No, we're selling the house, I'm living with Attia for now and then we'll see. Maybe I'll rent?' Said Tariq taking a sip of his drink.

'And what are you two doing?' Amit Bai asked Misha and Tushki.

Tariq answered for them 'they're in the States living with their mother.'

'I want to be a singer in Bollywood.' Tushki butted in.

'She sings well like her mother.' Tariq said proudly.

'Is Melia still working for the World Bank?'

'Yes, she just finished her Phd in physics at Stanford University' said Tariq grimly.

'She's a genius.' said Amit Bai.

'Yes, she's very clever.' replied Tariq filling up his glass.

'When's she coming back?'

'I don't know Amit, I just don't know,' replied Tariq, gulping down his drink.

'Baba you drink too much,' said Tushki. Tariq ignored her and took another gulp.

Two other girls walked into the room. One had cropped hair, the other a long plait. They led them to the table where the food was laid out. A man drifted by, Attia didn't introduce him. He was too well dressed to be a servant.

'Who's he?' Ana asked Mina.

'That's Attia's husband,' Mina whispered back.

Mina didn't understand. Why wasn't he eating with them? Why was he skulking around the house like a stranger?

They married young. It was a love marriage but Attia's parents never thought he was good enough for their brilliant daughter. Over the years the resentment built up as Attia excelled at medical school and her husband stayed at home doing nothing. She became the main earner, but even though she was a doctor she barely scraped a living. The strain was too much and they became estranged. Society would not tolerate divorce so they lived under the same roof for the sake of the children.

It was only after her husband left the room that Attia's face relaxed.

'More dhal … a little salad … please take some more,' she said.

As they ate, Ana sneaked glances at Misha and Tushki. Misha had long hair, shaved completely on one side and he wore a T Shirt adorned with a painted skull. His sister's hair was cut in a fashionable bob and her nails painted red, although she was Rimi's age. American school educated they both had thick twangs in their accents.

'Misha, do you think you will settle in the states or Bangladesh?' Asked Amit Bai.

Misha gave Amit Bai a quizzical look and said 'What do you think?'

Tariq was embarrassed and said 'I would like him to settle in Dhaka but there are more opportunities in the states. I mean I could have stayed in New Jersey. I had a big house, I was earning good money but Bangladesh is my home. This is where I belong.'

Attia's daughter started to laugh 'you're such a romantic. Bangladesh is finished. The government's totally corrupt, you don't get anywhere in this country if you don't bribe and there's absolutely no infrastructure. It's totally hopeless here. If I could get a visa to the states I'd be on the first plane out of here.'

Attia agreed with her daughter, 'she's right Tariq. If I'd accepted bribes I would be earning much more.'

Tariq grew vexed 'Of course there are bad people, there are bad people everywhere but there are also many honest, hard working people in this country.'

'Yeah, in the villages,' sniped Attia's daughter.

'No, that's not true. My workers in the textile factory, they were honest.'

'Yeah and look what's happened to the factory, it went bust,' Attia added quietly.

Tariq's eyes glazed over and he stopped talking. Amit Bai tried to change the subject and when Amit Bai talked the tension in Tariq's voice eased. They reminisced about the naughty things they did as boys in Barisal, drank whisky and everything seemed bearable and he forgot about his estranged wife, his ruined career and his hand to mouth existence.

The real Bangladesh

Trapped in a sandwich of baby taxis, buses, cars and rickshaws a woman with a long plait weaved through the mess of traffic on her moped. She zoomed past a man sitting on a chair in the middle of the bustle. He stared at his reflection in a mirror nailed to a tree with his face frothed up waiting to be shaved. Vendors arranged frilly dresses and bright things on the dusty floor. The driver was humming to 'Saturday Night Fever' as they paused by a flashing neon sign. A man knocked on Ana's car window, his forearm dangled from his elbow, boys thrust handfuls of pretty red flowers in Bela's face and the driver shooed them all away. They cut a corner and entered a side street. A kid was pissing in a steaming rubbish dump, a stray cow feeding off a pile of rot, a man carefully chiselling a face out of wood and a legless girl was sitting in a cart being pulled by another. They stepped out the car. Ana saw a low ceiling place where flies fed off silver fish and orbs of light shone out the darkness, a flock of cows, with skin ruptured from too many beatings, a shoemaker deconstructing an old shoe, a man pulling a cart of cauliflowers and another hammering in a dusty pathway. Amit Bai was taking them to see his big brother who lived in Paikpora, a place where the rickshaw drivers lived in shelters and slept on hard wooden benches. A place where Ana's nose swelled with the stink and her head grew dizzy with the haggle.

A middle-aged man with spiky black hair and lines of white in his sideboards was waiting at the iron gates. He hugged Amit Bai tight and said hello in strange high pitched English.

They climbed up several flights of stairs to a modest flat. Waiting for them was Amit Bai's brother, his wife and their many kids. On the table were dates, peeled orange, puffy rice, chickpeas, star fruit and pale green olives. Amit Bai sat close to his big brother. His teeth were all gone and the whites of his eyes yellow. His brother's wife watched them eat with careful eyes, filling up the plates every two minutes. She tried to make them feel welcome with dates, star fruit and olives.

'Take, take,' she said piling up Ana's plate with half a dozen.

Amit Bai's nephew, Mustak warned, 'don't eat too many, you'll get diarrhoea.'

His mother ignored him and slipped Ana some more. After the simple meal Amit Bai and Mina sat back, relaxed and chatted in the small living room. There was nothing flash about this flat. There were no pictures on the wall and no fancy rugs.

Mustak took them upstairs to the roof because he wanted to show them the real Bangladesh. In the pale light they saw the lines of squares, squiggles and blocks of black that made up the view. A woman hanging out her washing, enjoying the cool of the afternoon, a boy pushing a wheel twice his size and two men walking arm in arm. They could hear a baby crying, a man wailing against a backdrop of purple shadows, wooden shutters, and a patch of pink silk. From their humble perch in Paikpora they saw it all.

Ana looked up into the sky. It started off as a mighty rumble then it became a painful groan and the rain came down in fat pelts and it wouldn't stop. It just rained and rained and the sky changed from gold to black in less than a minute. The wind bullied the trees and slapped the heads of palms. Ana noticed a silhouette with eyes on her and crows were swarming low. It felt like just the start. Ana was standing in a world of light, dust, garbage, cockroaches, sweat and the wet puddle that was Bangladesh

GUNGI BLUES

Moustaches and rotten teeth

On their last day at Conna's house, Mina distributed gifts: a dressing gown for Mezu Kalu, A Talk to the Flower dress for Ellis and two bras for Conna. Mina had repaid their hospitality; she owed them nothing and could leave with a clear mind.

Mezu Kalu drove them to Boo Boo's flat in Cantonment. Her husband Boro Kalu was also a military general but they didn't have military guards with rifles. Boro Kala greeted them at the door. Amit Bai had told them that 'Boo Boo was beautiful. She was Nana's favourite because her skin was so fair.'

The lady standing in front of them had black thinning hair, a moustache, puffy eyes, a powdered ghostly face and a sour mouth. There was no hint of past beauty in her face. She smiled at Ana and patted her on the back with strained civility. Mina went to hug her sister but Boo Boo held back. She asked Mina 'Did you get the Fade Out' and Mina produced a large jar of the cream. She needed it to erase her age spots. She inspected the jar carefully and for a moment she looked happy.

Boo Boo led them all to the living room, snapping at the servant to make some cha and ordering her to put the Fade Out in the fridge. A tall man, with black shoe polish dyed hair like Mezu Kalu, walked in. Amit Bai leapt up and they did the back slapping ritual. Boro Kalu insisted on speaking English so that the children could join in. He was articulate, using words that Amit Bai didn't even understand. He proudly showed them a newly published volume of poems written in English. Ana noticed that the paper was the texture of recycled toilet role and the pages bound with grey string. Mina wasn't paying attention. She was too busy staring at Boo Boo. She could see that she wanted to talk to her but the words refused to come. Four young adults entered the room and Boro Kalu proudly introduced his kids. Neela, Sheila, Julie and Shaghor, the only son. They all looked completely different. Neela's skin was sherbet white, her face long and her toes even longer; Sheila was the colour of Marmite with thick wavy hair, Julie was a shade of milky coffee, short, podgy with a round jolly face and Shaghor was a creamy fudge, tall and slender with chiselled features and thick black hair. Neela and Shaghor had barely arrived before they had to leave. Julie was busy running after Tisha, her young daughter. At five years old Tisha had brown teeth and incipient gum disease from a combination of refusing to brush her teeth and eating too many sugary things. Julie lamented the fact that 'Tisha won't have any teeth by the age of ten.'

Ana looked over to Amit Bai who only had four teeth left. His front tooth was long and stained. The other two lay on the bottom jaw. Somehow that dominant tooth gave the impression of more teeth and Ana watched it protrude mightily in people's faces. Rimi asked Julie 'Where's your husband?'

Julie leant over and whispered in her ear 'Mintu isn't welcome.'

'Why not?'

'Abba and Amma don't like him because I ran off with him when I was sixteen. They think he ruined my life, they don't think he's good enough for me?'

'What does he do?'

'He's a musician.'

Julie pulled out a photograph from her handbag and Rimi saw a pale skinny man with a hooked nose and moustache. He looked like an Arab Inspector Clouseau. Julie stared at the picture fondly before placing it carefully in its special handbag place. Boo Boo was shouting at Tisha for leaving her lollipop on the carpet. Tisha just wiped her sticky hands on the sofa and ran off. Julie sighed

'She can't tolerate Tisha because she's dark. She's so strange like that.' Julie started to get emotional,

'Neela's married but she's childless. It's not her fault she can't have ... you know. They tried to marry Sheila off to a Bengali man in Sweden but she divorced him and now Abba ...' Julie restrained herself and said

'I'm sorry, you're so little, I shouldn't be telling you this.'

Rimi replied 'I don't mind.'

Jayida, who was far too beautiful to be a servant with her big eyes and smooth skin, called everyone for dinner. At the table Julie tended to the whims of Tisha, Sheila only ate rice balls and Mina and Amit Bai pretended to listen with interest as Bora Kalu droned on about his dream to be published in England. The food was worse than Mezu Kalu's spread. There were over cooked vegetable dishes, malnourished chicken legs and dry rice. The only dish that appealed to Ana was the cucumber salad. Ana reached out for some but Sheila said 'the cucumber is for Amma.'

Boo Boo was not at the table. Her bedroom door was slightly ajar and she saw her sitting on the bed with a needle in one hand. Ana nudged Bela to take a look. Boo Boo plunged the needle into her arm, powdered her face, added bright red lipstick to her pale lips, re applied her powder and then, only when she was satisfied, did she come out. After all her effort she looked like a ghoulish apparition.

Boo Boo counted the chapattees one by one and ate all the cucumber. She didn't seem in the mood to talk to anyone and during the middle of the meal Boro Kalu left the table and returned dressed in a white suit and blue shirt, made his apologies, went on about some urgent business meeting and left.

Boo Boo hissed something to him in Bangla as he whizzed through the door and they finished the meal in silence until they heard the shrill cries of a cat being raped. Boo Boo got up and went to her room. After a few minutes Mina followed her in and Ana heard the low murmur of chatter escalate into a more heated exchange. Amit Bai told Ana and her sisters to go outside onto the roof to play. It didn't seem to matter that it was pitch dark outside. Sitting in the gloomy flat was not much fun either. Sheila was studying in her room, Julie, Neila and Shaghor had gone home and the cats were still at it. As Ana and her sisters climbed the stairs up to the roof the shrill cries of the cat intensified and they started to giggle. Rimi thought they ought to go back to the flat but Bela wanted to watch. They stood in the doorway and observed a ginger cat humping a sleek black female from behind. Her paws were stretched out, her head flailing as she screamed in agony.

They walked into their parents' room to find Mina and Amit Bai lying in bed whispering to one another. Mina looked upset and Ana said 'What's wrong Mummy?'

Eventually Mina broke down 'Bora Kalu is having an affair. He wants to re marry but Boo Boo won't give him permission.'

Amit Bai told Mina to be quiet but she was unstoppable.

'She wants to throw her out on the streets because he can't stand her. She's sick, she has diabetes and she's not beautiful anymore, that's why he can't tolerate her.'

Amit Bai told Ana to 'go to bed and don't tell anyone this.'

As Ana brushed her teeth she watched a furry brown caterpillar pop out from behind the sink and tried to make sense of it all

The following morning Ana woke up to the sound of crows, lyrical prayer and whirring wheels. Boro Kalu was watching TV and cycling at the same time. Ana had never seen someone wearing a lungi on an exercise bike before. Jayida was sitting by the bike polishing his shoes and talking softly to him. Bora Kala walked in and told Jayida to 'go into the kitchen and start making the chapattees.'

Boo Boo turned off the TV and light leaving Boro Kalu in darkness.

'Are you mad? Turn it back on woman,' he yelled.

Then Boro Kalu saw Ana watching from the doorway and changed his tone. Smiling, he asked 'Are you hungry? Jayida heat some milk.'

Cracks of strain broke through his smile and although he clung on to a desire for normality there was the stench of madness in the air.

For the rest of the week Ana observed Mina following Boo Boo around the flat, hungry for a snippet of conversation but her sister was withdrawn and when they did talk it ended in a squabble about something trivial like the mess of bras, dirty cotton buds and entangled saris in Mina's room. Amit Bai told Mina 'Not to bother.'

Despite being constantly rebuffed, Mina couldn't help trying. But Boo Boo's life consisted of a strict routine. At nine am a cleaning lady came to wash the floor, at ten Boo Boo watered her plants, at eleven thirty she sat on the roof to sun her legs, at twelve she supervised Jayida to kill a chicken, at two she took her injections, at two thirty she had a nap and woke up at four in plenty of time for Boro Kalu's return at five, they ate at six, he left the flat at seven and then she watched TV until eight and went to bed alone. Everyday was the same and there was no room for Mina.

Boo Boo spent most of her life cooped up in the flat brooding. She barely exchanged words with her daughter Sheila. Ana's cousin didn't seem to mind preferring to stay behind closed doors and memorise Sociology books. Her other children did not bother to visit. When Shaghor occasionally walked through the door, her face lit up and she promised

'I will send you to the States, you don't have to worry about money.' Shaghor was her shining light.

She had been married thirty years to a man who was having affairs and there was nothing she could do about it because she was totally dependent on him. Boro Kalu provided the servants, insulin, gold bangles and clothes on her back. She was forced to endure her farce of a marriage because walking away was simply not an option. And the bitterness built up inside her. She still looked at herself in the mirror, still rubbed lotions in her skin, still saw herself as beautiful and she couldn't understand why Kalu didn't want her anymore. Beautiful Boo Boo. All the men in the village were after her and now her life had come to this. Some days she didn't want to live but suicide was not an option so she terrorised the servants and snapped at her kids. She could no longer tolerate seeing her husband, knowing what he was up to, knowing she was powerless but she had to stay put because she had nowhere else to go.

GUNGI BLUES

Keys

Mina said 'we're leaving at two thirty' and told her three children to sit down for lunch. The room was swimming with people. Boro Kalu was proudly showing Amit Bai a new publication. Julie's daughter was running around the table, her stick thin legs were covered in bites. Sheila was hiding behind a book in the corner. Neela was trying to persuade Mina to part with a flower patterned handbag and the three children sat at the table looking at plates. Boo Boo called everyone for dinner but there was no time to enjoy the food. Boro Kalu kept reiterating 'their car will be here soon,' but Boo Boo argued 'there's no rush let them eat,' and filled Ana's plate with rice that she didn't want.

'They'll miss the ferry' Boro Kalu snapped.

Boo Boo ignored him and piled a dollop of meat curry onto Ana's rice. As she raised her hand to stop the influx of food, Ana noticed there was a faint glimmer of a smile on Boo Boo's face. And the frown that never seemed to leave her forehead had definitely softened; a sign of relief perhaps that her five guests were finally leaving. After a mouthful of food they filed downstairs to the car. Sheila waved from her seat; she didn't bother to get up. Neela had disappeared and Julie was on the phone but she flashed a sweet smile at them before returning to her chat. Boro Kala and Boo Boo came downstairs to see them off. Mina and her sister exchanged a few words and Boro Kalu said proudly, 'next time you come you can stay in my new house; it will be five stories high with a pharmacy downstairs. It's not built yet but I've already bought my plot of land.' No one was really listening to him. They were too busy squeezing into the car. Amit Bai shook Boro Kalu's hand through the car window, 'come to Manchester' he said and Ana wondered if Amit Bai really meant it.

They left the spacious quiet of Cantonment and within minutes they were back in the heart of Dhaka city. Ana looked out and saw half-completed structures propped up on bamboo sticks and hand-painted billboards for Fair and Lovely soap. A woman gathered sticks in an ally way. Forty people hunched up in a tiny van. A family of six piled into a rickshaw. A beggar tapped on a car window with his stump. A cow snorted rubbish in a field. An old man, with scraggly white beard and ravaged chocolate face, peddled his rickshaw. A double-decker red bus bombed past him, it was jam-packed with people. They stopped at the lights trapped in a thick line of traffic. A boy was slashing the ground with a pickaxe. He was one of many boys heaving concrete slabs into place. Beside him was a man sleeping face down in the dust. Hidden in the shade of twenty tyres. Walking by was a woman with a red tangle of hair and a face covered in a smudge of ash grey. In her arms she carried a sleeping baby and its tiny brown bum peeped out at Ana.

GUNGI BLUES

They left the heap, the huddle, the stench, the dust, the heat and sweat of Dhaka city and entered the leaf, the light and water of Burigongi River. Water hyacinths sat still on the water. Houses on sticks balanced precariously on the edge. Two men played chess by the side of the road. Children played cricket in a paddy field. Chunks of field were sliced up into quarters. The trees watched a man plough his field in the smoky light. And Amit Bai shouted at the driver to 'hurry up or we'll miss the ferry.'

They reached the port just as the ferry was pulling out to leave. It was an hour until the next one. Ana stepped out with her sisters. The light was pink, the water calm, people smiled and stared. Everyone's eyes were on the three girls. Bela and Rimi stuck to Mina as she haggled over the price of a bunch of bananas. Amit Bai and the driver stood on the water's edge watching the ferry chug by. Coward that Ana was she retreated into the air-conditioned comfort of the car. The driver returned and asked 'Do you want to listen to music?' Ana nodded.

'Eagles or Bee Gees?' He asked.

Ana was soon shaking to the grooves of Saturday Night Fever and watching people from the safety of the car. To her left a man was slicing papaya into small squares, which he bagged in polythene and placed in a basket. He did not waste any flesh. His daughter was sitting beside him. Her hair was cropped short, eyes blackened with eyeliner, lips painted red, legs covered in scars, feet worn and older than her years. Her father grunted at her and the girl smiled as she lifted up her dress and removed a handful of taka stashed down her green underpants. Her father stuck the money in his shirt pocket, wiped his knife clean and placed the basket of papaya on his head. The girl slipped under the shack behind her and pulled down her pants for a pee. She returned, readjusted her green knickers and took a swig from a battered plastic bottle. Then she sat down and stared at a forlorn goat that walked by. To Ana's right were dark skinned, bright eyed, white teethed boys selling hard-boiled eggs in baskets. A man lit a joss stick, sipped on a bottle of Coca Cola and spat. A squinting blind girl wandered with an outstretched palm. She eyed a bunch of browning bananas hanging overhead and a man shooed her away like a fly. In the distance Ana saw a man in a white vest, muscle bound with glistening chocolate skin. He oiled up a pan and fried chapattees one by one. It was dark now. Light bulbs shone out from stalls cluttered with crisps, peanuts and cigarettes. A long line of men walked by the car carrying bundles on their heads, sucking on fags. Ana felt a twitch in her left leg and opened the car door. She stepped out for a second, making sure to lock the door behind her. Eyes pounced on Ana and she quickly walked back to the car, tried to open the door but it didn't open because it was locked from the inside. Ana tried another door and another but they were all locked. And then she saw them. The keys dangling from the wheel and Ana wailed in a mixture panic and shame. Within seconds people crowded the vehicle and Ana's skinny body was squashed against the car. They were everywhere, faces, hands and people shouting 'why did you get out of the car.' Ana searched around. Where were the nice little boys selling eggs, the papaya man and the blind girl? Where were they now?

The driver came over, saw the keys in the car and raised his hands to his head. Amit Bai started to shout at Ana: 'what have you done you bloody idiot?'

'I'm sorry ' Ana said 'I didn't mean to.'

Mina, Bela and Rimi came over, all munching on bananas. Rimi looked anxious, Mina asked 'What's going on?' and Bela offered Ana a banana.

'Why did you lock all the doors?' Amit Bai shouted.

'I don't know' Ana said.

'Go and wait over there.' He said with a look of disgust.

The three of them sat in a nearby Tea House. It wasn't really a Tea House. It was a decrepit place with cheap plywood floor, news papered walls, blue plastic nailed to the tables, rough benches, dirty plates stacked high and blackened toes. A man offered Ana a small cup of tea. She took a sip. It tasted like liquid sugar. As they waited people stopped and asked 'who are they?'

The chapattee man relayed the story and people laughed, pointed and stared. Ana closed her eyes and wished she was somewhere else, back in Manchester in her bedroom playing with Lego. She re-opened her eyes and saw a man opposite, eating sloppy rice. Ana turned away and saw three young men standing in front of them. 'Bangla boley.' They asked. 'Hey Bangla boley' Ana pretended she couldn't hear.

One man caught Ana's eye. He was looking down at his dick and smiling. His friends started to laugh. Ana felt sick. Rimi grabbed Ana's hand and got up to go. Bela wanted to stay, Rimi pulled her away but there was nowhere to escape to. People were still crowded around the car sticking pieces of wire into holes with little success. Amit Bai was itching his head, Mina looked fraught and when he saw them standing by the car he shouted 'I told you to stay inside. Go on.'

Amit Bai managed to call Dhaka from the Tea House and two hours later a tired man arrived with a spare set of keys. A young man tapped Ana on the shoulder and said that the 'Car's open now.' Ana ran past him and dived into the car. 'Staying Alive' was blasting out and Amit Bai snarled 'turn off that damn music'

Ana didn't care because suddenly she felt safe once more.

It was ten pm; they'd been stuck in this hole for five hours although it seemed much longer. The stars were bright in the Dhaka sky and eye of the moon stared down at Ana sternly. Ana would have liked to have spoken to the moon if the moon could have spoken back to her. When she blinked, the moon blinked and shined a little brighter. It was time to sleep but to sleep would have been a colossal waste when the world was awake and there for the taking.

The air was humid, the sky a reddish black. At first it was quiet and then the sky began to rumble and churn. The wind fought with the trees and millions of rain droplets spat down on the car with contempt. Ana watched the people sleeping in lopsided boxes by the roadside and the odd foot stuck out resting on a mattress of dirt. An old man squatted under a weary looking tree; his head was hung well over his knees. He didn't have a bag of possessions, he didn't have any sandals, he didn't have anyone. All the outcasts of Dhaka society began to converge at night. The driver got out the car and bought some cigarettes. He rolled one in between his forefinger and thumb. Then Ana opened the window of the car and watched her hair dance in a spurt of wind. The driver parked the car by a back street lit up with oil lamps. He parked in a discreet corner and told the three children to keep their head low. 'It's dangerous here, bad people here.' He told Ana.

Bela interjected 'I want to get out.' 'Why?' The driver asked ''Just to see' Bela replied. The cab driver gave her a quizzical look and lit up a cigarette. Bela and Ana slid down and watched the play unfold. It looked like any back street with oil lamps and people milling around, most of whom did nothing but stare and loiter. Women began to appear wearing bright saris; some were old and young, fat and slender. They wore thick red lipstick and strange blue eye shadow. A young mother nestled her baby close and kissed its forehead repeatedly before handing the child over to a small boy barely twice the size of the baby. The clients were wrapped in checked, faded lungis. Dishevelled, dirty, undistinguished types, like vendors or local rickshaw drivers. They couldn't have paid more than a few taka a pop.

Skulking in the shadows were a couple of transvestites, skinny men with a full face of make up wearing saris. It was like a freak show. Undetected, Ana watched until one young lady in a bright red sari with a gold embroidered edge walked over and tapped on the driver's window. Amit Bai waved a dismissive hand. She didn't notice the three children. The driver eyed her up and then emulated Amit Bai. Ladies led man inside low-level huts. The men re-emerged ten minutes later followed by the women who counted the taka and then looked up anxiously for more customers. There was one girl, she was tiny like a doll, she looked about eight but she was probably twelve. Malnutrition made these girls slender and fragile.

GUNGI BLUES

Her eyes were lined with black kohl and her smudged red lipstick was too garish for her delicate mouth. She didn't look afraid, she didn't look fearless, she just looked blank. The girl sat down on the ground and rearranged the orange carnations that garnished her neck. Men were looking at her and she looked back and smiled. It was at that point that Ana wanted to leave not wanting to watch her go into a dark, damp hut, not wanting to imagine. The beautiful child had equally captivated the driver; perhaps if he'd been alone he would have paid for one night with her?

The ferry arrived and within a few minutes Ana turned her back on the child, on that world of lipstick and blue eye shadow and drove away.

Cockroaches and silk

Seemed like they had been travelling forever. Tired, hungry and dirty they finally arrived in Barisal. It was four am, too early to wake people up. So they parked up by the side and waited. Ana needed to go and squatted by a wall for a pee, half fearful, half asleep, half awake. She heard footsteps. A man walked by and paused to spit. Then prayers boomed out and Ana couldn't escape that ancient chant. Ana stumbled through the dark and climbed back in the car. Amit Bai looked out the window at his house and started rambling

'You'll meet my father today. He was the first ever graduate from Dhaka University you know. He is so patient and calm. He always helped me with my maths homework. He never shouted when I didn't understand my sums.' He said fondly.

The children stayed quiet and wondered why Amit Bai shouted at them when they got their sums wrong.

Mina was subdued. This would be her first meeting with Amit Bai's parents. She was nervous. In their eyes she was the woman who lumbered their youngest son with three kids at twenty-seven, depriving him of a fresh bride and clean start in life. How would they feel towards Bela, Rimi and Ana? They were not their real grandparents; they were no relation, just strangers.

GUNGI BLUES

Amit Bai led the way into the house. Ana banged her foot on the ridge and banged her head too. Amit Bai rang the bell and a shrivelled lump of a lady opened the door and she embraced her son like a long lost precious thing. She started to cry and whisper Allah's name over and over. Her hair was like white silk, her eyes wide and deep black.

'Ashu, ashu' she croaked ushering Amit Bai in with a veiny hand. Her feet were a tiny size three her toes slightly wrinkled. A man with rotten yellow teeth and white curly hair was eating his Shahari. He was Amit Bai's brother; his wife stood by and looked at everyone with dead eyes.

'Say hello to your Phu Pha and Cha Chi.'

Phu Pha and Cha Chi stared at the three girls strangely. Perhaps it was because Bela and Ana were wearing identical BHS velvet jogging suits with floppy hats and red open toed sandals.

'So thin.' Cha Chi said looking at Ana. She shrugged her shoulders and smiled as she watched a cockroach crawl on the table and hide under a pan.

'Where's Abba?' Amit Bai said anxiously.

'He's waiting for you in there,' said Phu Pha with his mouth full of rice.

An old man sat in a room sparsely furnished with two wicker chairs and a small side table. The walls were stone, patterned with cracks and discoloured with age. The man sat, slightly tilted to the left, his hand rested on his right knee, his heavy belly sagged between his checked lungi and his brown sandaled feet were turned out. On his head he wore a furry hat that looked like an upside down cup case. His mouth was framed in a dignified pout. A neat white beard sprouted from his chin and his green eyes searched out for his son. 'Amit' he croaked.

Amit Bai ran like a little boy to Dada and then he called the children in. 'Go on.' He said.

'Salam, koru' said Amit Bai losing patience.

Rimi was the first to stoop down and touch Dadu's tiny toes; she did the same with Dada who patted her head gently. Ana copied her big sister. Bela was next in line but she hid in the kitchen refusing to kiss anyone's feet

Amit Bai. Dada and Phu Pha stayed in that room and Phu Pha's loud chatter drowned out the soft flow of Dada's voice as Amit Bai tried to listen to his father.

The children followed Dadu up a stone flight of stairs. She took them to a room with pale blue walls and a stone floor. Clothes were piled in a bulk, boxes stacked under the bed and a blond curly haired doll stood in a pink box, on the dressing table, waiting to be opened.

Kettles and Elvis

Dadu put up a mosquito net as the three girls struggled in the dark to find their pyjamas. The bed was hard, the pillow stiff, the air thick with heat and the singsong of crickets that kept Ana awake until six. Ana sneaked out from under the net and felt her way downstairs to the bathroom. She opened the door and saw a room with a tap, a bucket and a jug. The walls were stone and the ceiling covered in a web of mosquitoes. Ana undressed slowly. Her socks were the last to go. Reluctant toes touched wet stone and Ana washed in cold water as fast as she could, longing for hot baths in Manchester. Ana felt the mosquitoes pierce her skin, she swore and slapped the thin air but they still got her. Then Ana heard a croak of a voice and a knock.

When Ana opened the door she saw Dadu holding a tiny kettle. She thrust it in her hand and turned on the light switch. 'Thank you very much' Ana said and poured the warm water over her toes. She could hear the fizz of bubbles in her ears and saw soapsuds on her knees but she didn't rinse, didn't even dry her body, just stuck on her clothes, undid the latch and scurried out. Dadu was waiting for Ana again. She offered her a banana and Ana munched on the sweet thing as she investigated the house. The kitchen was papered in newspaper. The walls were a flaking blue and sepia. Outside was a ditch inhabited with monster plants and a knotted tree. The water was covered in a thick layer of green and rubbish. To the right was an old wooden door that stood out against an orange wall.

GUNGI BLUES

Ana pushed the door open and saw a pink toilet set in the ground. To the left was a shack made of corrugated sheets. Ana returned to the kitchen and wondered why there was a poster of a non-descript woman hanging on the wall. She pushed another door and saw gigantic stone pots huddled together in the dark. Chinks of light crept into murky corners and guided Ana to a stone flight of stairs. Red checked lungis blew in the breeze, sucking up the sun, hanging from lines strung out on the landing. Ana glimpsed Phu Pha and Cha Chi sleeping in separate beds. Phu Pha slept with his mouth open and Cha Chi's curled up body seemed to blend into the leaf pattern of her bedspread. Dusty fat books, that had turned brown with age, lined uneven shelves and a chair basked in luminous patterns of light. Ana climbed up a second flight and reached a final door, pulled it open, stepped out on the roof where she saw slender trunks dressed in changing light and a woman washing pots in a pond cluttered with too many trees and squiggles of bush.

Fifteen minutes later a young woman with thick curly hair and a broad backside appeared, shielding her face from the glare of the sun.

'Hello, I am Liana your cousin.' She stared at Ana and cooed 'you're so pretty' and started to caress Ana's head with gentle fingers.

'You have so little hair,' she said in stilted English.

'Do you colour it?'

‘No’ Ana replied.

‘Are you hungry?’ she asked and returned with strong tea and biscuits.

‘It’s so hot. Your face will burn and your skin will turn black.’

‘I don’t mind,’ Ana replied. ‘I really don’t.’ Liana shaded her face with an arm that was covered in spidery hair. Her skin was pale. Pale from years of avoiding the sun by sitting in darkness.

She sighed and said ‘you’re too young now but one day you’ll get married like me.’ Then she ran off and moments later she emerged with a giant size wedding photo in which her face was perfectly painted and she was dressed in gold and red silk. ‘Do you like?’

‘Yes’ Ana lied.

‘This is my husband’ she said producing a blurred passport photo in her palm.

‘He’s thirty-six. Ten years older than me. Do you think it’s too much?’

Ana shrugged her shoulders thinking how ugly the man was.

'He is in New York. He's a doctor. I will join him in America. He says that if the marriage doesn't work out we can split. I like him but I do not love him. How can I? I spoke to him twice on the phone, we married and then he returned to America.'

'Aren't you going to live with him?' Ana asked

'Yes in three months. I like America. I like Elvis Presley and Fleetwood Mac. Do you like, also?'

Before Ana could reply Rimi and Bela appeared with Mina and Munni the maidservant. Munni was a tiny girl with a big smile. She carried a bucket of water and a bowl full of wet washing. Mina instructed the three of them to sit and to bend their heads low. She poured water over their heads and lathered their hair with Vosene shampoo in the blaze of the sun. Bela squealed 'I've got soap in my eyes.' And Ana protested 'I already had a wash.' But Mina didn't seem to hear.

Three small children watched from the opposite rooftop, vaguely amused. Munni hung out white sheets and when Mina had finished washing her hair, Ana escaped downstairs with Liana.

Pomegranate and Jesus

Lianna and Ana squeezed into a rickshaw. She wore a sparkly Salwar Khameez and carefully painted lips.

They passed rickshaw drivers mending punctured tyres, men welding in the street, tiny stalls selling fruit, sweet houses and barber shops. Ana saw a boy sitting in the barber's chair, draped in white cloth. His pea head was bent forward waiting for the clip. Ana saw a church made of red brick and Bengali priests donning white robes. Lianna took Ana beyond the iron gates and they strolled down paths and enjoyed the spacious grounds. They saw a woman looking through a barred gate, the cool stone interior of the church, elegant archways and men plucking grass. They reached a lane that led to a house. A woman with a weathered face invited them in and offered them sweet orange squash and thick biscuits. They sipped on the sweet drink and noticed a picture of Jesus Christ on the wall. They left the quiet still of the church and returned to the street, stopping off to buy Roshaguli, pomegranates and grapes. They past a cow, a man carrying a pole, thirty foot long and a fading shell of a house. Finally, they reached Amit Bai's house. Munni was still hanging washing and a man, wearing bi-focals, sat cross-legged hacking at a coconut. Dadu was sitting in the doorway on a low wooden stool. Deep in meditation she didn't flinch she just swayed a little now and then before getting up to go to the bathroom. Bela and Rimi were drinking Tomato Cup A Soups in the front room. Amit Bai and Mina had gone out with Dada. It was two o'clock in the afternoon and Liana's mother was still sleeping and Phu Pha was listening to the cricket standing up. Ana roamed the house and got a shock when she saw Dadu half naked in the bathroom. Her hair was loose and cascaded in wisps of white down the sagging folds of her ancient body. Ana said 'sorry' and gently closed the door.

Moments later, shrouded in white Dadu was sitting on the bed, head bent over that green holy book, rocking back and forth. She let the light warm up her legs and wiggled her toes in concentration. Ana heard the gun gun of her chant and didn't want to disturb her.

'Go on' coaxed Liana 'Give them to her.'

Swallowing her inhibitions, Ana offered the brown paper bag of fruit to the old woman

Dadu looked in the bag and muttered 'I've got no teeth'

'You can suck on the grapes' said Liana gently. Dadu reflected for a moment, took the fruit and patted Ana roughly on the head.

She stashed the bag by a wall of stuff hidden behind a thin cloth. Stuff collected over decades. Then she sat sucking on grapes, spitting out pips. Glad for the sweet change. She looked up at Ana and offered her the pomegranate. Ana took it not knowing what to do with it. She shouted for a knife. Munni came running with a small machete. Dadu squatted, happily engrossed and taking a knife in her bony hand she hacked off the hard shell. She peeled and pulled with fingers. Red beads of fruit sprayed everywhere, mostly on the floor. She offered Ana a handful of the red shiny things. Ana took the beads of fruit from Dadu's wet, wrinkled fingers and ate. There was a mess of skin and splinters of red on the floor. Ana watched her struggle to scoop up the slippery peel. Offered to clean up but she said 'I can do it' and told Ana to sit down and 'eat,' She chucked a handful of peel out the window into the ditch clogged up with years of debris and returned to her grapes. Ana sat opposite Dadu with a bowl full of pomegranate; sweet and juicy Ana guzzled down the whole lot. And as she stuffed her face Ana watched her toes, tiny and delicate in their wrinkled perfection. Watched the way her hair fell across her face. Examined the hard, worn bed on which she lay. The stone floor on which she rested her feet, the barred windows, the dim green neon bulb that jutted out the wall and the knackered sideboard. How could she live in this one hundred year old pit?

Ana tried to imagine when she was younger. Amit Bai told them how he ran away from home one day. He was supposed to be circumcised. When he finally returned Dadu beat him with a stick. Somehow Ana couldn't picture this frail lumpy thing with her tiny fingers and toes, instilling fear of any kind and Ana stayed for a while fixated on those toes.

Dadu started to arrange, shift and fiddle. Looking slightly agitated she said,

‘I have to pray now.’

Ana took the hint and got up to go. Dadu stopped Ana with a tug of the arm and dumped another helping of pomegranate in her bowl, then she shooed her away with a bony hand and Ana left.

A Visit

It was a balmy afternoon and Mina was taking a nap. She was feeling calm. Dadu and Dada had welcomed them. They never mentioned Ravi; they never brought up the past. Bela didn't make life easy by refusing to say hello or thank you and insisting on only drinking Cup A Soups and eating Sugar Puffs but Mina could live with that.

Munni entered Mina's room without knocking.

'Babi, there's someone here to see you', called Renu.'

'Who?' said Mina straightening her plait.

'She says she's Ravi's sister or something.'

'What?' Mina panicked. How did she know they were here and what did she want? Mina frantically brushed her hair, changed into an elegant sari and called the three girls into the room.

A slight lady, the spitting image of Bela walked in. After inspecting the three children up and down she asked in Bangla 'Mina how are you?'

'I'm fine.' Mina adjusted her sari when it didn't need adjusting to avoid making eye contact. The lady was staring, making Mina twitch.

'Your children are very beautiful'

'Why have you come here?' Mina was getting agitated.

Renu started to laugh, sat down on the bed. 'Why have I come here? To see my nieces of course, they are so pretty especially this one' she said smiling at Bela but Bela didn't smile back.

Mina was struggling to keep calm and the lady sensing a tinge of hostility changed her tone. 'There was something I did want to talk to you about.' She sighed and paused to choose her words carefully.

'Times are really tough now. I'm in a financial mess. It was terrible after Ravi died.' She said looking down at the floor.

'He used to send us money but when he died you cut off contact just like that.'

She looked Mina in the eye now 'we are short of money when we shouldn't be. It's not right we are entitled to part of Ravi's estate, as his wife you're not entitled to a single penny.'

Mina's nostrils flared and she fired back, 'do you think we are made of money or something? All we have is 6 Whitebrook Road. If we give that up where are we supposed to live, on the street? Look how much do you want?' Mina said directly. 'I have five thousand taka, take it.'

'I don't want your paltry taka, I'm not a beggar.' She snarled back.

'Just take it?' Renu took it but she didn't seem grateful.

'I didn't really come here for money. I really came because I want your daughters to meet my boys. It's what Ravi would have wanted.'

'I'm sorry.' There was a deep frown cutting Mina's forehead in two. Renu seemed in her own world and waffled on 'your daughters should marry my boys, they're in their twenties. They'd make perfect husbands. Not now of course but in a few years.'

Bela and Ana were only kids and Rimi hadn't even started her periods yet.

Mina exploded. She didn't shout she spat out her words one by one in a voice that made Ana tremble. 'Are you mad? Look at them. They're little girls. I think you'd better leave now.' Mina's eyes were glazed over and Ana thought she was going to cry.

Munni came running into the room

'Show her out please.' Said Mina in a broken voice.

Renu left looking bewildered and Mina collapsed on the bed. Ana went up to Mina and asked 'Who was that woman?

Mina remained mute curled up in bed with her arms wrapped around her head. That frown stayed with her for the rest of the day, cutting into her skin, giving her a headache. How could that woman come here? She thought. Who told her they were in Barisal? She hadn't come to say hello. She didn't care for her kids, she just wanted to marry them off to her stupid sons. Just wanted Ravi's bloody money. Mina was suddenly glad she'd left Bangladesh all those years ago. Glad to escape people like this. And she longed for the quiet of Manchester and the calm of her own bed.

Beautiful Sun Rise

Everyone was sleeping and Ana was on the roof, the sun was not yet up, the light soft and hazy. Sleepy rickshaw drivers peddled down the lane. Men with heads wrapped up in scarves paused to cough up phlegm. One man saw Ana standing in her pyjamas and she backed away. The air was damp with dew and Ana shivered as she tried to watch her sun rise. A girl burst through the door, squatted and took a pee. Turning away in embarrassment she disappeared leaving a wet trail behind her. The sun finally burst through with the burn of its rays. What a sunrise. Ana had never seen light that pure before. She tried to take it all in one last time but a black crow swooped down on the ledge and intimidated her into leaving.

Ana roamed the house for the rest of the day. Noticing things that others didn't see. The metal rusting beams, the Mona Lisa print in the hallway, the unmade beds, the bottles of Fair and Lovely on the dressing table and the Horlicks jar filled with Rich Tea biscuits. Munni was picking through a basket stacked with green leaf. She got up to check on her fish shiny with fat. Dinner was ready and they all sat down to eat. There were not enough chairs so Phu Pha ate standing up. Lianna de-boned Khoy fish and offered some to Bela but she was happy with a bowl of Sugar Puffs. Rimi was too scared of the bones and Ana stuck to rice and dhal. Amit Bai and Mina had two helpings of Khoy, sucking and chewing the bones into purple piles of pulp. Dadu and Dada ate sloppy rice. Cha Chi was still asleep. And then it was time for them to leave. Everyone walked them to the door. Ana took one final look at the house. Walls hadn't seen a lick of paint in a century. Garden had never been pruned, trimmed or mowed. Giant pots never been used. Old tin cans left to rust. Damp left to mould. Stone left to crack. Neglected for one hundred years, it was still beautiful in its crumble

Las Vegas

They arrived at the bus station; it was crowded with too many people everywhere and waited in a room with a TV set. An Indian drama blasted out to keep people entertained. After half an hour of waiting it was time to board the bus. There was hardly any room but they managed to squeeze on. There was a smack of Las Vegas about Bangladesh with the buildings showered in neon lights, even though they were dilapidated and small. Then Ana saw a limbless beggar rolling down the streets on a skate board, another with a grossly inflated leg and an old woman with wrinkled polythene skin sitting by the road. After a while Ana grew bored, closed her eyes and tried to sleep on Mina's silky lap. Mina put down an Asda carrier bag to stop her dribbling on the silk. Ana tried to get comfy but it was impossible with the constant jerking, spitting and coughing in her ears. By five they reached the first stop; a stop where they could brush their teeth. The coach parked up in a squalid place, dotted with kiosks, the ground was lumpy with broken stones and mud. Beggars just pounced on people as soon as they got off. Mina carried a polythene bag of one-taka coins that she seemed to give to everyone. Amit Bai guided the children to some 'clean toilets,' the stench was unbearable and the sound of coughing relentless. They were soon back on the road munching on a breakfast of apples and greasy fried chicken, weaving through narrow dark lanes that felt like sinking black holes.

GUNGI BLUES

The coach pulled up and two skinny men started to unload the luggage. People flocked, poked and prodded in search of their own cases. Amit Bai spotted theirs and escaped the scrum. Hailed two rickshaws and made their way past peeling soft peach and pale lemon buildings; past people dragging carts three times their weight; past people making rice in the street; past boys selling pomegranate juice; past a dried up girl selling silver elephants; past a boy spitting at his father; and past a mad man with dreadlocks sleeping in a home made of string. They stopped by an uprooted tree. Must have been hundreds of years old. It lay with its roots in the air like a woman showing her knickers to the world.

In the distance was a pink house with a wooden roof. A young girl was slapping slop onto the ground and a pale old man with a long white beard was supervising her. When he saw the five of them arrive in the rickshaws he cried out Allah's name and raised his hands in the air. Mina just looked into her father's eyes. How long had it been? This was the first time she'd seen him in years. She still remembered the day she left the house. He had stood there with tears in his eyes unable to look at her, unable to say goodbye. Too much had happened in between. Nothing shared. Nothing said for too long. If Nana felt any sadness now he hid it well. Perhaps he was happy to see his grand kids and Amit Bai. There was a bright something in his eyes but his smile was weak. He looked Mina up and down and the first thing he said to her was 'you've gone dark and put on weight.' Then he turned to the three girls and said proudly 'But your children are fair.' And stroked their heads.

Mina was frowning and there was a moment of silent staring before Amit Bai hissed at the children to Salam. They followed Nana into the house. It was cool and dark with shutters drawn and lights switched off. Nana opened the back door and there was a girl sitting on a battered sheet of plastic.

'She's Dilu, the servant's daughter.' Said Nana looking at the girl fondly.

Her feet were bare, her hair oiled up and her face covered in a mask of snot and dust. The light spread into warm purple shadows on her skin. Four puppies sat in her lap. She pulled at one pup's ears and flicked its' nose. Then she raised her hand and smacked it on the head, once, then twice until it ran away. She picked up another, gripped it by the neck, swung it in her tiny hands and threw it to the ground. Chickens were pecking at rice. A small woman was brushing her teeth with a finger. The little girl's father was washing from the stone basin in the yard and a bitch was licking her teats. Ana watched, hidden behind a towel on a washing line that reeked of damp. Saw curious faces watching her from behind the fence. She went back inside, examined the delicate watercolour on the wall and a photograph of a man who looked familiar. His skin was soft, his glasses big and his eyes deep. The sight of a spider stuck to the wall made Ana flinch and she could almost feel the creep in the shadows.

Nana wanted to take them to see the town. Mina let Bela and Ana go, there was not enough room for Rimi, she stayed behind and helped unpack. Nana didn't talk much but it felt comfortable sitting next to him. Everyone seemed to know him. He waved at people who asked 'who are they?'

'They are my grand daughters; they live in England.' He said as if this was something important.

During the ride they saw women in colourful saris carrying plates of sand on their heads'. They were working on a building site of cement mixers and bricks. Further on they passed a decrepit white temple, its garden was over grown, its grounds deserted. Ana noticed a man taking a bath behind a thin screen on the street. There were two rickshaw drivers, one was a young boy whose feet barely reached the pedals, the other an old man with a gaunt face and long white straggle of a beard, both struggled with the weight they had to pull. They reached the Bazaar and watched workers fry Gelapi in hot fat. Flies sucked on stacks of brown, pink and yellow sweets. Men sat on the floor selling mountains of oranges. A cow's head lay in the dirt, its limbs swung from hooks swarming with flies and the three men chatting nearby didn't seem too bothered.

Nana took them to the river. People were crossing the other side in slender boats. The banks of the river were covered in thousands of stones hand laid one by one. Ana looked into the water. It gleamed like silver but it stank like shit. An old man took off his clothes and disappeared under the water, others washed clothes, some bathed, and even swam. A little further on they discovered hills of green tea planted years ago by the English. Spindly trees, with white painted trunks, gave shade to the women walking by in red, purple and green. They followed them down camouflaged paths that lead to narrow streams and more leaf. Occasionally someone emerged through the bush with baskets hanging from poles slumped against tired shoulders. They left the bush and travelled to a place where Queen Victoria may have sipped tea once upon a time. Stared at the green valleys and watched the shadows lengthen with the setting sun. It almost could have been somewhere in England.

GUNGI BLUES

Billy Bert and Fred

When they got back Nana left them alone to explore the chickens, geese and three silky goats tied to a tree. Slim and sleek they went up to say hello and Bela christened them Billy, Bert and Fred. Stroking them Bela whispered sweetly in their ears. Nana came out to offer them warm goat's milk that tasted like lumpy puke and said 'you can play with the animals as long as you want. This is your home. Feel free'.

Ten geese congregated in a corner and looked docile enough. Bela approached them for a closer look. Within a second their long necks swooped down and they went for her legs. They ran back into the yard and found a wicker lid lying on the ground. It was moving ever so slightly. The three of them hovered over the lid, desperate to see what was underneath. Bela didn't hesitate and lifted it up. Ten fluffy yellow things came running out in all directions. They tried to gather them up but the chicks went mental and slipped out of their hands like wet bars of soap as they tried to grab them. A big black crow swooped down and snatched one up. A second came from nowhere and nabbed another. Nana came out when he heard the commotion and quickly gathered as many as he could. In the end they lost six. Nana said 'don't worry, play with the goats instead.'

Bela became very attached to Bert and plumped him up with long grass and leaves all afternoon. By six o'clock Nana returned with three other men. The men untied Bert, Fred and Billy and guided them to a grassy verge. One of the men was sharpening a knife on a slab of stone. Another looked like a holy man with his string of beads and funny hat. Nana was smiling and told the three girls to sit down and watch. The holy man began to mutter under his breath and Billy was pulled forward, his head stretched back as the man sliced his neck with the knife. The blood began to seep out in trickles and then splattered out in all directions. Billy bleated helplessly and his eyes rolled in his sockets. Rimi turned away and Bela glared at Nana. Billy's skinny legs collapsed and he fell to the ground with a soft thud. They watched his body being dragged away. His glossy skin was covered in dirt and his tongue lolled out of his mouth. Fred, a shade of brilliant white, was next in line. He fluttered his eyelids not knowing what was in store for him. The man came up from behind and attacked his neck with the knife. Fred jerked as a wasp flew up his left nostril and missed the flying blade. Grasping him roughly by the ears the man went for his slender neck again and this time slit it deep. Fred fell to the ground. His white coat was soaked in brilliant red. Bert, the most beautiful out of the three, with his big brown eyes and droopy ears, was pushed to the bloody mud patch. Bela started to cry. Crying was her only form of protestation and she wouldn't stop. The knife came down and hit the bone. Bert bleated in shock and writhed in pain as he squirmed and kicked in an attempt to break free. The man pulled out the knife and hacked once more plunging the knife into Bert's flesh. A jet of blood shot out and Bela screamed as Bert dropped to the ground in a mess of blood, goat and mud. It was all over in less than ten minutes. Nana looked over and smiled but he saw the disgust in the three faces. He couldn't understand. He had sacrificed the goats in the name of Allah, they should have been happy. Ana, Bela and Rimi wanted to see Billy, Bert and Fred one last time to say good-bye before they were buried but they couldn't find their hacked up bodies. Despite the stench, they sat in the mud patch littered with goat droppings. That's where Billy, Bert and Fred had been standing only half an hour and they sat there until the mosquitoes started to bite.

The following day they lost themselves in the forest at the back of the house and temporarily forgot about Billy, Bert and Fred. The forest was a place that engulfed you, extending far and deep and there was a wooden toilet placed there thoughtfully for roaming kids. In the afternoon Rimi bathed in the pond, just as Mina used to when she was a kid, while Bela and Ana sucked on sugar cane, cuddled chicks and taunted geese. Nana was either praying or out somewhere, Amit Bai ate like a pig and Mina sat by the pond, gazing into the water and trees like a deranged hippy from the 60's. They had been at the house for two days and Ana had barely seen Nanu. In fact Ana hadn't once seen Nana and Nanu together as a married old couple. They seemed to coexist in separate spaces, Nana in his room, and Nanu in the small mud hut kitchen at the back of the house. Most days Mina sat with her mother.

She didn't say anything, just watched her move. Seemed content to just sit with her mother.

The smell of roasted rice and toffee drew Ana towards the kitchen one morning. Nanu appeared in the doorway shrouded in a veil of steam and handed her a round sticky thing. It was still warm; Ana took a bite and said 'thank you very much.' They stared at one another because that's all they could do. She couldn't speak English and Ana's Bangla was substandard. There was silence. Silence Ana wanted to fill with silly chatter. She discovered traces of Mina's cheekbones, deep-set eyes, fat lips and snippets of herself in Nanu's face. That was the closest Ana got to her.

On their last day Nana came into the bedroom and spoke to the three girls in long mellifluous sentences, almost like prayer. He talked about Allah, urged them to be good Muslims and told them that 'I pray for Allah to be with you and your mother. I've always prayed for you and your mother and you must pray for me and write to me when you get back to Manchester'

He broke into prayer and began blowing on Ana's face, over and over again smothering her with the stale odour of his breath. He repeated the ritual with each of them. Then they loaded their stuff into a rickshaw, waved goodbye and Nanu handed them a plastic box with carefully sliced papaya and a plastic bag of apples and oranges. As they rode down the shady lane, past thick walls of tree and those crumbling peach walls, Ana wondered if she'd ever see the little pink house in the middle of the bush again, with its nasty geese, its emerald pond, its fat forest and its Billy, Bert and Fred.

The Gate

It was their penultimate night in Bangladesh. Tariq was throwing a little party to say goodbye. People sat politely on sofas sipping on whisky including Mina and Amit Bai. Only Tariq sat cross-legged on the floor and started to sing in a tipsy voice. Tariq wanted his big sister Tulu to come but she stayed at home. Tulu was his favourite out of his sisters. She was the one who listened to his problems, who gave wise words of advice about his failed marriage to Melia, who maintained the precarious balance between warring factions. She relished the role of mediator, counsellor, and peacemaker. Tulu spoke in a soft voice that betrayed the temper that belied her round cheeks, kind eyes and silky elegance. Tariq loved to shout over any minor incident. 'Where's my hot water you bastard?' 'This food tastes like shit.' He would rant. The servants were no longer offended by his outbursts because they knew it was just hot air, frustration and pain. The pain he was still suffering after his wife Melia left him for a Pakistani man in New Jersey. Pain from the pressure of maintaining the pretence that Melia was still his wife that she still loved him and was coming home.

Tulu lived in Gulshan with her daughter and their maidservant. Just the three of them. The maidservant's name was Mohua. Most of her adult life revolved around Tulu and her daughter Aveen. Whenever they needed her she was there. Didn't have to shout twice. She ironed, cooked and cleaned. Mohua was attentive and 'caring' they said afterwards. Perhaps over caring, over concerned, over interested. Asked too many questions, hovered in the bedroom to watch over her Aveen and Tulu. They were her only family. And after ten years of loyal service she was their equal. She could read and write she was no different from them. Circumstance had made her the servant.

Mohua was chopping green leafy stuff with a thin blade. Cutting it swiftly and deftly with the same knife she'd used for the past ten years. It was still sharp although the metal blackened and the handle worn. Aveen and Tulu were sitting at the table waiting for dinner. The table was bare apart from two glasses of water and Mohua was in no hurry. Pots simmered and farted out wisps of steam. It would all be ready in another ten minutes. There was still the salad to prepare, the coriander to wash, the chillies to chop.

'Mohua' Tulu yelled impatiently, Mohua came running with the knife still in her hand,

'What's taking so long?'

'Another ten minutes,' she smiled showing off her red stained teeth.

'Another ten minutes, we've already been waiting twenty. Just bring out the food.'

'But I only need ten minutes' Ten minutes for her final touches, then they could feast on her soft aloo, spicy Khoy fish, fluffy rice and hot dhal.

Groans of hunger from Tulu's belly drowned out Mohua's pleading. She didn't like the way Mohua answered back. She should have just obeyed. That's what servants were supposed to do. There was no discussion. Tulu's was the final word.

'Mohua, just bring the food out right now.' Mohua was about to argue but Tulu stared at her.

It was a deep stare. A stare that left her cold like a swallowed ice cube, a stare that made her feel small like a tiny ant in the desert. A stare that opened the rusty gate previously locked for years. There were many occasions when Mohua bit her lip, cursed the saucepan and kicked the bitch that begged for food scraps. The gate, which Mohua had kept safely locked was suddenly open for the first time. Like a river breaking through flimsy barricades, Mohua found herself sitting in the kitchen shaking with anger battling with a tirade of feelings that she couldn't fathom. Tulu was hungry; she wanted her food right now. Tulu had been waiting twenty minutes and the rumbles in her tummy were growing louder. That's all. But why did she feel insulted, bruised and battered with a heavy pan. Why did she feel resentment deep and thick like glue? The knife was still in Mohua's hand. Her palm was wet with sweat. Her grip on the knife tight like fingers strangling a fragile neck. Mohua emerged. Her heart was pumping. She could feel it throbbing through her red sari blouse. She tried to speak but the words wouldn't come. Too choked, too entangled, too buried in something. Tulu glared at Mohua 'Where is the food? I told you to …' Tulu grew silent as she watched Mohua walk up to her with the knife by her side. The edge of the blade curved up like a silver crescent moon and glinted in the light. Aveen saw a strange glazed look in Mohua's eyes. 'What's wrong?' Tulu asked quietly.

Mohua didn't hear the question. She was facing Tulu and in one bold sweep, like cutting the head of a chicken, she sliced away Tulu's cheek. A surreal moment suspended in time. Almost like slow motion. Tulu's screams didn't put Mohua off. Aveen was paralysed in her chair, stuck in shock. Mohua hacked and hacked at her master. Hacked at her like a tough loin of beef. Swiped at her bare arms, her waving hands, her flailing head until she was unrecognisable. Parts of her lay about on the marble floor, a finger, cheek, hair, flesh, blood. Tulu was now a collection of small bloody parts on a bed of shredded red silk. Tulu could no longer give her a headache with her shrill screams because she was dead. Aveen was shaking in her chair realising that if she didn't escape she'd be next. Mohua and Aveen had always been close, like sisters she thought, Aveen ordered her around a little, took Mohua for granted, shouted at her almost daily but only for minor things. Mohua was the servant, it was her job to be shouted at. Aveen had done nothing wrong, Mohua would spare her. Aveen looked down at her murdered mother. One eye was still open. Frozen in an expression of disbelief. Mohua looked up at Aveen and smiled. She stood up and walked towards her. Aveen tried to smile back but incipient fear made her mouth twist up into a grimace, or perhaps a derisive smile, or perhaps it was disgust. Mohua stared at Aveen's eighteen-year-old pretty face. Her fair skin, her thick black curls, her shapely figure. Aveen was disgusted with her and Mohua didn't like it. Never liked the fact that Aveen corrected her spelling and her grammatical mistakes. Never liked the fact that Aveen could speak English fluently and had only taught her to say 'bowl'. Found it annoying that she had so many friends, was so adored and so sickeningly perfect. Hated the fact that Aveen was going to Dhaka University to study English, and would probably marry a handsome rich man and leave her alone to rot by herself. Mohua lunged at Aveen. She jerked out of the way and went running to the door. Mohua always double locked the door at night so that nasty intruders couldn't break in. Aveen tried to pull open the bolt that only Mohua had the strength to open. Aveen never liked to touch the bolt because the metal was always shiny with grease. The bolt refused to budge as Aveen wrestled with it. She suddenly felt the shadow of Mohua behind her. Silent and soft. Felt the blade sink into her back. A sharp pain made her knees collapse and fall to the floor. Mohua leant over her. How beautiful she looked now with her hair shrouding her shoulders and her brown almond shaped eyes fluttering their pretty lashes at her.

GUNGI BLUES

Aveen screamed 'Please, please, don't do it.' Mohua chopped off Aveen's hair until there was only an inch left like a sprouting of fresh grass. Aveen's chest heaved up and down, her generous breasts peeping though her blouse. Aveen watched the blade rise and fall across her chest. Blood squirted into Mohua's face like a spat out insult. Mohua couldn't stop. She began to carve a pattern of lines across Attia's body ending with a final cut to the neck to plug the screams pouring out the hole of Aveen's mouth. Silence filled the house now. Mohua sat on the marble floor observing the blood pools, wondering if they would stain, she'd better clean it up before it ruined the good marble, before Tulu had a go at her. Tulu's dismembered body seemed to have melted in a thick pool of blood. Mohua got up and stood over her once podgy mistress. She gently kicked her head and laughed. Laughed because she was kicking her mistress's head without fear. She walked into the kitchen and closed the door. Washed her blade clean until it looked like new once more. Changed into her best sari and sat down to eat her sumptuous meal, the meal that they could have enjoyed too if they'd been bothered to wait for ten minutes. She ate all the food, quickly as if she knew that someone might come. She ate until the skin of her stomach stretched tight over her bulge. And then she put up her mosquito net and went to sleep, sound and deep.

Mohua gave herself up the next afternoon because she was tired of waiting for someone to come and discover the bodies. Secretly she wanted to see the horror in their faces. She wanted the handcuffs, the intrigue, and the questions. But no one phoned, no one came by because it was the day when people slept in and picked their feet. Mohua watched the flies feast on an ear, an open eye, and cakes of flesh. Where did all these flies come from? They must have travelled miles, driven by the smell of sweet meat. The flies covered the bodies in a moving black shroud, licking, eating and feasting. Mohua began to feel nauseous from the stench. She got changed. Used Aveen's blusher to give her dark cheeks a pink tinge. Combed her hair with Aveen's ivory comb. Even put on one of Aveen's best saris, yellow silk with a purple flower patterned border. She peered at her reflection in the full-length mirror. Aveen's white-heeled sandals gave her an extra couple of inches, making her body look slender. How slim she was? How pretty? She had even features and smooth skin. If only she was fair like Aveen. Then someone would want her. The face Mohua saw in the mirror was an eighteen year old, fresh with the bloom of youth. Now she was forty-eight and looked quite ridiculous with her over painted face and clothes too bright for her years. She had been married once, at nineteen, but her husband died of pneumonia. They hadn't been married long enough for love to form, to make babies and go on rickshaw rides. His sudden death forced her to find servant work. Forced her to find any way to survive.

She left the house, making sure to lock up, and walked proudly down the street on her way to the police station to give herself in. There were no handcuffs, not that many questions and no intrigue, A prompt trial two months later and four damp, dark walls for life. Mohua didn't see the walls; she only saw red marble and the open gate that led to the garden. A garden with grass, and leafy Deb Daru trees, a garden where she could lie and sleep in the open air, a garden where she was free.

The papers said that Mohua had viciously killed Tulu and Aveen in an unprovoked fit of rage. They'd had a row but Mohua couldn't remember what the row was about. Neighbours heard the screams but they didn't intervene. Just thought they were having a domestic, like most people did.

When Tariq was told 'your sister and niece have been murdered' the day after the leaving party, at first he didn't register the words. Mina couldn't believe it either. She didn't know anyone who had been murdered and never thought she would. Mina took her three daughters to one side and quietly said what had happened. It was a story that Ana was not quite sure how to respond to because it seemed so unreal. Their last day in Dhaka was sombre and Ana couldn't wait to return to Manchester to escape the details of hacked off ears and fingers.

Each year Tariq and his relations gathered on the day of Tulu and Aveen's bloody death and prayed.

Prayed to Allah that they were in heaven somewhere. These gatherings were supposed to unite the family, stop the bickering and ease the familial strain. But nothing was said during these gatherings. Just prayer, chat and tea. Everything that they really wanted to say lurked within, gasping for air but was kept shut inside for years just as it had been in Mohua. Trapped behind closed gates, waiting.

GUNGI BLUES

Black Eye

Their flight was at four am and Dhaka airport was eerily deserted. The sun slowly rose and flooded the departure lounge. They were finally leaving Bangladesh and Ana felt a strange affinity and revulsion at the same time. She longed for rainy old Manchester, the orange buses and the smell of her bed, but Ana wanted one last ride on a rickshaw, a final suck on a stick of sugar cane and as she squinted in the rays of the rising sun she knew she'd miss that special light.

Landing at Manchester airport the first thing Ana saw were traces of snow dressing patches of green; the last remnants of winter. They shivered in the taxi home, and looked out the window at the drab greyness. Saw a dirty orange bus and an old aged pensioner standing at the bus stop. It started to rain and people got drenched. There wasn't a trace of blue in the sky and the sun was smothered in grey cloud.

6 Whitebrook Road had grown into a semi mansion in Ana's imagination. Now accustomed to spacious living rooms and double beds when Amit Bai opened the front door the hall was disappointingly tiny, the kitchen cramped, the living room a box. Where were the servants and the chauffeur? Amit Bai walked into the kitchen put on the marigold washing up gloves and attacked the pans that had been left to soak in dirty water for a month. Tomorrow Ana would be up at seven to get the 172 bus to school. On Saturday they'd buy baked beans

at Asda and in the afternoon there'd be hoovering and Jim'll Fix It if they were good.

That night Ana dreamt of Billy, Bert and Fred. She even heard them bleating in the night. It wasn't bleating that Ana heard it was the cries of Amit Bai, a scuffle and a sudden thud

Two men, one white, the other black, broke into the house. One of them smashed the glass, slipped in his hand, unlatched the door and stepped into the kitchen. They cleaned out downstairs within five minutes and made their way upstairs. Mina's bedroom door squeaked as it opened. She opened her eyes. Amit Bai was snoring. She could hear rough breathing in the air. Then she felt a hand on her hairy leg; cold and clammy. She screamed out. That's when Amit Bai got out of bed and started to shout incoherent things. The man shot out the bedroom door. Cursing them in Bangla Amit Bai followed them downstairs into the hall. There was no contest. Both six foot they towered over Amit Bai; he was only five foot four. Amit Bai continued to shout at them in Bangla until a flying fist shut him up. He fell back onto the stairs and the two men darted out into the night through the front door. Amit Bai got up straight away and called the police. They said they'd be there in five minutes. He sat on the stairs waiting for them with a bag of frozen peas on his black eye. They came three hours later. By now the thieves had probably flogged the video, telly and Hi Fi but Amit Bai gave a statement anyway and even made the policemen a cup of tea.

GUNGI BLUES

Mina couldn't sleep for a week after the burglary. She didn't feel safe in her own bed anymore. She kept on dreaming about cold fingers and in the end that was the reason why they finally left 6 Whitebrook Road and moved to the posher part of Manchester.

Eyes open 1999

Ana opened her eyes after reliving the memories of her first trip to Bangladesh and sat in the tiny spare room by herself. Ana still remembered how ashamed her parents were that they didn't speak Bangla, she remembered the curious stares and the comments, she remembered the strange sounds and the light that warmed her soul. That was the only time they visited Bangladesh as a family. It was reassuring for Mina to see that Conna and Boo Boo were equally dysfunctional. That madness infected their lives, irrational behaviour and curious ways. Grown up now Rimi, Bela and Ana were scattered in various places. Rimi was in Barcelona, married to a spliff smoking, multi lingual Belgian, Bela was a single mother, living on benefit in Devon, Ana was a struggling artist, living in London and her parents were stuck in Manchester with their memories and dreams. They resembled two innocuous dumplings, incapable of instilling fear of any kind. Bela had long forgiven Mina for the beatings. she understood what it was to be a parent; even her own son had screamed 'I wish I was adopted.' Bela concluded that 'they screwed up but that doesn't make them monsters.' Mina was carrying so much stuff inside she wasn't aware when it started to 'leak' – that's how Bela put it. Did it matter now anyway, Ana was an adult? It was all in the past. Did it matter that Mina was a psycho at times? Weren't all parents like that at some point. Did it matter that she still didn't understand what it meant to be a Muslim? Did it matter that her Bangla was still crap. Did it matter that Mina had posed for in the nude. Wasn't that proof of her mother's love.

Mina's squidgy body

When Ana looked at her mother's body she saw soft flesh and pillow breasts. Nipples like saucers and travelling veins. Elegant fingers and wiggling toes. A tremendous black pitted arse. Rough bits and smooth bits. Hairy patches and sparse pubic hair. But no cellulite.

This was Mina: beautiful and grotesque. A fascinating landscape that at first Ana was too scared to explore. She was the one who didn't need much persuading when Ana tentatively suggested that she draw her in the nude. Mina always wanted to be free like a bird. Flashing her black bottom at inappropriate moments. Singing out of tune and dancing around in skimpy, lacy things. And when she stood naked in front of Ana it was she who was embarrassed and looked away. She sat proudly squeezing her droopy boobs together and Ana looked down. She told Ana to hurry up please because she was getting cold and the postman was coming. Ana fumbled with her stump of lead and tried to avoid her eyes. She was giggling now like a little girl and then she was grumpy, asking Ana why she made her do such awful things.

It was Amit Bai who first proposed the idea, over Sugar Puffs, one Sunday morning.

'Ana, you should draw your mother full naked!' He spurted out excitedly.

Ana was stunned for a second but then monumental nudes of Mina flashed in her head. Those same glorious images invaded her dreams, and still did, but something frightened Ana. This was her mother. Ana felt pangs of guilt at what she had done to her delicate cheek bones, almond eyes, button nose, pink shapely lips and her lush, squidgy body. When Ana turned to her mother for approval she said that in all honesty she didn't understand what she was doing and probably never would but if Ana was happy she was happy and that's all that really mattered.

The garden

A sound made Ana get up, it was still dark. She looked out and saw Mina, squatting on a stump in her night dress and wellies. Mina was gazing out into space flashing a torch light. Ana didn't know what she was looking at. 'Those leaves need pruning and that needs weeding. I'll do it later' Mina said to herself. She was watching Robi, her pet rabbit. The black and white furry thing she named after Rabinranath Tagore – the Nobel Prize winning writer. Secretly Mina believed the spirit of Tagore inhabited her rabbit. She could just tell by the way he chased cats and gorged on Rhododendrons. 'He'll eat my Clematis next' she thought as Robi dived into a shrub but she didn't budge from her stump.

Amit Bai never wanted a rabbit, Ana didn't see the fascination either, they seemed like rather pointless creatures that lived for grass, humped slippers and twitched their nose a lot. But Mina wanted one. She wanted a rabbit to live at the bottom of the garden in a hutch by a little wooden house just big enough for one. A place where she could hide away and watch the sky at night. Amit Bai bought the little wooden house, the rabbit and a gold fish. The fish committed suicide but the rabbit got fat, lived on and ran wild in the garden.

What was this place she had created with its trees, its corners and its shady hidden bits? 'It's my Pahtuakali jungle' Mina said. It was her bit of Bangladesh brought home.

GUNGI BLUES

The garden wasn't a place with neat borders, trimmed grass and colour co-ordinated shrubs. It was a place to get lost. It started off with a round patch of grass that seemed to shrink under the weight of the climbing Honey-suckle, the minty spotted Laurels and wild Montana. A path of chipped bark wound into another place shaded by a massive Sycamore tree. There was a small Willow by the fence, which used to be brown but it was covered in three-toed Ivy now. A bench lay hidden around the corner, a place to sit and watch dancing Campolinas under the Yew tree. Heavy with red berries it spread itself like a tent over the garden. There were juicy pink things, furry stems, blue sky flowers, snake patterned leaves, sweet golden roses, velvet petals, pink elephant ears, furry lamb's tails, bell shaped blooms, Fuchsias that spread like quilted purple skirts and Bamboo shoots ten feet tall. Ana remembered the garden when it was a nondescript patch of grass, with weeds and feeble borders. She remembered when it was just another rectangle with nothing much going for it. She remembered when it was a mess. Full of shapes, smells and strange things, this was Mina's landscape now, the place for her imagination to run wild, and the place where no one could tell her what to do.

Ana ventured out in search for her mother and heard music coming from the house at the bottom of the garden. A sweet voice, a flute, a subtle tabla beat. She edged closer and saw Mina was no longer on her stump, she was lying on her back looking up through the window. Her arm was wrapped around her head, her forehead stuck in the crease of a stale memory that wouldn't go away. Was she thinking about her dead husband Ravi? The one who haunted her. The one she saw everyday. Was she thinking about her mother? Was she thinking about her children, that Ana was too thin and Bela too mad? Mad like her. Was she blaming herself for the way they'd turned out? Was she blaming herself for not being the mother she wanted to be whatever that was? Beside her was a cup of hot water dipped with onion. She read somewhere that it cleared up a blocked nose. Her face looked calm for once. Her toes were twitching to the beat. She caught Ana watching her and all she said was

'You know I'm from another planet, I'm just visiting, I'm waiting to go home.'

Ana didn't understand. She couldn't even pretend to. What did she mean? Which planet was this? Which other world was she talking about? Ana didn't know.

Epilogue

Bangladesh was like entering another world. Alien, beautiful grotesque, scary, smelly and quite breathtaking all at once. It wasn't a place Ana could relax, feel comfortable or warm. It wasn't a place she could shout or take a walk to the corner shop. It was just the place where Ana's parents were born. Ana was born in Manchester. Bangladesh was a place to visit, to discover and learn but never to live. To live there would mean their crumble. Forced to hide behind white powder, tight lips, strained silence or thin pretence they wouldn't know how. Manchester was their home. It wasn't perfect but that's where they lived, that's where they could be whatever the hell they wanted to be.

And Mina and Amit Bai might dream of living in some distant land that was warm with clear blue skies with water far and deep but wasn't that everyone's dream? Amit Bai had his Ford Mondeo, his house, his pension. And Mina had her memories of Nana and Nanu. Memories of a childhood that left her warm and cold, that let her melt into dreams but she could always wake up. And when she woke up to the damp of Manchester in her king-sized bed, she saw Amit Bai snoring beside her. She heard the music of Eastenders downstairs and the tremors of a fight brewing. She smelt stale fish curry in the curtains. She saw old newspapers lying on the bedroom carpet, the broken duck on her windowsill, her little man made jungle outside and it was some strange comfort. It was some strange comfort to them all because this was the only place where they were really free. Free to act out their gungi ways and feel their gungi blues.

GUNGI BLUES